OSTEOPOROSIS

A Lifecourse Epidemiology
Approach to Skeletal Health

OSTEOPOROSIS
A Lifecourse Epidemiology Approach to Skeletal Health

Edited by

Nicholas C Harvey
University of Southampton
and
University Hospital Southampton NHS Foundation Trust
Southampton, UK

Cyrus Cooper
University of Southampton
and
University Hospital Southampton NHS Foundation Trust
Southampton, UK

University of Oxford
Oxford, UK

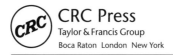

CRC Press
Taylor & Francis Group
Boca Raton London New York

CRC Press is an imprint of the
Taylor & Francis Group, an **informa** business

CRC Press
Taylor & Francis Group
6000 Broken Sound Parkway NW, Suite 300
Boca Raton, FL 33487-2742

© 2018 by Taylor & Francis Group, LLC
CRC Press is an imprint of Taylor & Francis Group, an Informa business

No claim to original U.S. Government works

Printed on acid-free paper by Bell & Bain Ltd, Glasgow

International Standard Book Number-13: 978-1-138-19616-2 (Paperback)
978-0-8153-7716-0 (Hardback)

Library of Congress Cataloging-in-Publication Data

Names: Harvey, Nicholas C., editor. | Cooper, Cyrus (Professor of Rheumatology), editor.
Title: Osteoporosis : a lifecourse epidemiology approach to skeletal health / [edited by] Nicholas C. Harvey, Cyrus Cooper.
Other titles: Osteoporosis (Harvey)
Description: Boca Raton, FL : CRC Press/Taylor & Francis Group, [2018] | Includes bibliographical references and index.
Identifiers: LCCN 2017042305| ISBN 9781138196162 (pbk. : alk. paper) | ISBN 9780815377160 (hardback : alk. paper) | ISBN 9781351234627 (ebook)
Subjects: | MESH: Osteoporosis | Osteoporotic Fractures | Risk Factors | Bone Development--physiology
Classification: LCC RC931.O73 | NLM WE 250 | DDC 616.7/16--dc23
LC record available at https://lccn.loc.gov/2017042305

Visit the Taylor & Francis Web site at
http://www.taylorandfrancis.com

and the CRC Press Web site at
http://www.crcpress.com

Contents

Preface

Osteoporosis is a disorder whose time has come. Recognised since antiquity (Figure 0.1), the impact of the condition through its association with age-related fractures, an understanding of its cellular and molecular pathophysiology, clarification of risk factors throughout the lifecourse, development of risk assessment algorithms to predict absolute fracture risk and the discovery of a wide range of effective therapeutic interventions which attenuate bone loss and prevent fracture, have led over three decades to a conceptual transformation. The ill-defined, poorly understood and inevitable consequence of ageing described in scattered monographs only 40 years ago has matured into a fully qualified member of the non-malignant group of noncommunicable disorders which will increasingly plague the cash-strapped healthcare systems of both developed and low/middle-income countries of the world as they deal with ever-increasing numbers of older people. This monograph addresses these translational innovations in our understanding of osteoporosis and integrates them into a lifecourse approach to prevention and treatment.

The term *osteoporosis* was coined by pathologists in France and Germany during the middle decade of the nineteenth century. The description was essentially morphologic, based upon reductions in both cortical thickness and trabecular architecture. It was paralleled by observations on the patterns of occurrence of fractures in older people during the post-Renaissance explosion of rationality as applied to the physical and life sciences. Thus, Ambrose Parey in France and Astley Cooper in the United Kingdom, both orthopaedic surgeons by clinical discipline, remarked upon the striking excess of hip fractures in older people, the relative excess of fracture rates in women as compared with men and the notable seasonality observed even at that time. Although they postulated a potential role for impaired bone strength in their aetiology, it remained for Fuller Albright, a senior endocrinologist at Massachusetts General Hospital in the mid-twentieth century, to link estrogen deficiency in postmenopausal women with reduced bone mineral density and elevated fracture risk. The subsequent demonstration that postmenopausal estrogen replacement reduced fracture risk, and that this effect was mediated by an inhibitory influence on osteoclastic bone resorption, led to a resurgent interest in the non-invasive assessment of bone density in

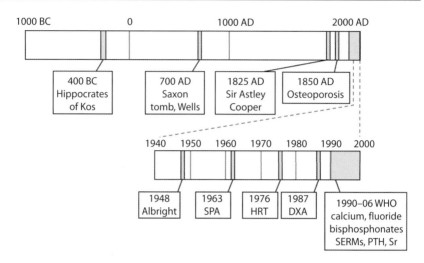

Figure 0.1 The evolution of osteoporosis as a disease across three millennia. DXA, dual-energy X-ray absorptiometry; HRT, hormone replacement therapy; PTH, parathyroid hormone; SERM, selective estrogen receptor modulator; SPA, single photon absorptiometry; Sr, strontium ranelate.

humans, and culminated with the launch of dual-energy X-ray absorptiometric bone mineral density (BMD) assessment in 1987.

The provision of this key intermediary biomarker of fracture risk permitted the World Health Organization (WHO) to define osteoporosis according to the population bone mineral density distribution (2.5 standard deviations below the young normal mean) in 1994, heralding the last quarter century of intensive pharmacologic innovation with release of a variety of anti-resorptive and formation-stimulating agents now available, including oral and intravenous bisphospho-nates, denosumab, raloxifene, teriparatide and abaloparatide. The last decade has witnessed the delineation of national and international strategies to target these agents most efficiently and cost-effectively at those patients who will ben-efit most (and are least likely to sustain the rare but important adverse effects) from these interventions. This personalised strategy, focused principally on those who have already sustained a fracture and those with important additional risk factors, has been augmented by a realisation of the lifecourse determinants of fracture risk. It is now clear that environmental influences during the earliest periods of intrauterine development, and perhaps even preconception, can alter gene expression through a variety of epigenetic routes and thereby modulate the peak bone mass attained by the end of the second decade of postnatal life, as well as the subsequent rate of bone loss. Coupled with lifestyle modification during childhood, adolescence, mid-life and old age, these discoveries open the door to a parallel population-based preventive strategy against fracture throughout the lifecourse. This volume attempts to integrate these innovations, to contextualise them within broader international attempts to combat musculoskeletal ageing and preserve physical function and to consider the most effective clinical guidance for employment of the newly developed risk-based strategies in routine primary and secondary patient care.

Cyrus Cooper
Nicholas C Harvey

Editors

Nicholas C Harvey, MA MB BChir PhD FRCP, is Professor of Rheumatology and Clinical Epidemiology at the MRC Lifecourse Epidemiology Unit, University of Southampton, and leads a world class programme of research on the lifecourse epidemiology of bone and joint disease. His work is focused on the translation of epidemiological observations linking early life influences with later bone health into potential novel public health strategies (e.g. gestational vitamin D supplementation) aimed at optimising childhood bone mineral accrual and reducing risk of later fracture; elucidation of underlying mechanisms; and investigation of novel risk factors for poor bone health in older age. He has won several awards at national and international meetings, is an investigator on >£50m grant funding and has published over 150 peer-reviewed papers. He is Vice-Chair of the International Osteoporosis Foundation Committee of Scientific Advisors, Musculoskeletal Lead for the UK Biobank Imaging Enhancement, and a member of the American Society for Bone and Mineral Research Professional Practice Committee, National Osteoporosis Society (UK) Scientific Programme Committee, UK Bone Research Society Committee, Arthritis Research UK PRC and UK NIHR Regional RfPB Panel.

Cyrus Cooper, OBE DL FMedSci, is Professor of Rheumatology and Director of the MRC Lifecourse Epidemiology Unit, Vice-Dean of the Faculty of Medicine at the University of Southampton and Professor of Musculoskeletal Science at the Nuffield Department of Orthopaedics, Rheumatology and Musculoskeletal Sciences, University of Oxford.

He leads an internationally competitive programme of research into the epidemiology of musculoskeletal disorders, most notably osteoporosis. His key research contributions have been discovery of the developmental influences which contribute to the risk of osteoporosis and hip fracture in late adulthood, demonstration that maternal vitamin D insufficiency is associated with suboptimal bone mineral accrual in childhood, characterisation of the definition and incidence rates of vertebral fractures and leadership of large pragmatic randomised controlled trials of calcium and vitamin D supplementation in the elderly as immediate preventative strategies against hip fracture.

He is President of the International Osteoporosis Foundation, Chair of the BHF Project Grants Committee, an emeritus NIHR Senior Investigator and Associate Editor of Osteoporosis International. He has previously served as Chairman of the Scientific Advisors Committee, International Osteoporosis Foundation; Chairman, MRC Population Health Sciences Research Network; Chairman of the National Osteoporosis Society of Great Britain; and past-President of the Bone Research Society of Great Britain. He has worked on numerous Department of Health, European Community and World Health Organisation committees and working groups and has published extensively (over 900 research papers; h-index = 119) on osteoporosis and rheumatic disorders and has pioneered clinical studies on the developmental origins of peak bone mass. In 2015, he was awarded an OBE for services to medical research.

Contributors

Bo Abrahamsen
Odense Patient Data Explorative
Network
Faculty of Health
University of Southern Denmark
Odense, Denmark
and
Department of Medicine
Holbæk Hospital
Holbæk, Denmark

Michael A Clynes
MRC Lifecourse Epidemiology Unit
University of Southampton
Southampton, UK

Juliet E Compston
Cambridge Biomedical Campus
Cambridge, UK

Cyrus Cooper
MRC Lifecourse Epidemiology Unit
University of Southampton
and
NIHR Southampton Biomedical
Research Centre
University of Southampton and
University Hospital Southampton
NHS Foundation Trust
Southampton, UK

and
NIHR Oxford Biomedical Research
Centre
University of Oxford
Oxford, UK

Elizabeth M Curtis
MRC Lifecourse Epidemiology Unit
University of Southampton
Southamptom, UK

Elaine M Dennison
MRC Lifecourse Epidemiology Unit
University of Southampton
Southamptom, UK

Mark H Edwards
MRC Lifecourse Epidemiology Unit
University of Southampton
Southamptom, UK

Mark Hanson
Institute of Developmental Sciences
University of Southampton
and
NIHR Biomedical Research Centre
University of Southampton and
University Hospital Southampton
NHS Trust
Southampton, UK

Nicholas C Harvey
MRC Lifecourse Epidemiology Unit
University of Southampton
and
NIHR Southampton Biomedical
Research Centre
University of Southampton and
University Hospital Southampton
NHS Foundation Trust
Southampton, UK

John A Kanis
Centre for Metabolic Bone Diseases
University of Sheffield
Sheffield, UK
and
Institute for Health and Aging
Catholic University of Australia
Melbourne, Australia

William D Leslie
Departments of Medicine and
Radiology
University of Manitoba
Winnipeg, Canada

Karen Lillycrop
Biological Sciences
Faculty of Natural and
Environmental Sciences
Institute of Developmental Sciences
University of Southampton
and
NIHR Southampton Biomedical
Research Centre
University of Southampton and
University Hospital Southampton
Southampton, UK

Namrata Madhusudan
MRC Lifecourse Epidemiology Unit
University of Southampton
Southampton, UK

Eugene V McCloskey
Centre for Metabolic Bone Diseases
University of Sheffield
and
Centre for Integrated Research in
Musculoskeletal Ageing (CIMA)
Mellanby Centre for Bone Research
University of Sheffield
Sheffield, UK

Michael R McClung
Oregon Osteoporosis Center
Portland, Oregon
and
Institute for Health and Ageing
Australian Catholic University
Melbourne, Australia

Rebecca J Moon
MRC Lifecourse Epidemiology Unit
University of Southampton
and
Paediatric Endocrinology
University Hospital Southampton
NHS Foundation Trust
Southampton, UK

Ruth Muller
Munich Centre for Technology in
Society
Technical University of Munich
Munich, Germany

Shane A Norris
WITS/SAMRC Developmental
Pathways for Health Research Unit
Department of Paediatrics
and
Faculty of Health Sciences
University of Witwatersrand
Johannesburg, South Africa

Michi Penkler
Munich Centre for Technology in
Society
Technical University of Munich
Munich, Germany

John M Pettifor
WITS/SAMRC Developmental
Pathways for Health Research Unit
Department of Paediatrics
and
Faculty of Health Sciences
University of Witwatersrand
Johannesburg, South Africa

Ann Prentice
Nutrition and Bone Health
MRC Elsie Widdowson Laboratory
Cambridge, UK
and
Calcium, Vitamin D and Bone Health
MRC Keneba, MRC The Gambia
Unit
Serrekunda, Gambia

Ego Seeman
Departments of Medicine and
Endocrinology Austin Health
University of Melbourne
and
Institute of Health and Ageing
Australian Catholic University
Melbourne, Australia

Kate A Ward
MRC Lifecourse Epidemiology
University of Southampton
Southampton, UK
and
Nutrition and Bone Health
MRC Elsie Widdowson Laboratory
Cambridge, UK

1

The burden of osteoporosis

ELIZABETH M CURTIS, NICHOLAS C HARVEY AND CYRUS COOPER

INTRODUCTION

Osteoporosis constitutes a major public health problem, through its association with age-related fractures, particularly of the hip, vertebrae, distal forearm and humerus, with serious consequences in terms of morbidity and mortality. Worldwide, osteoporosis causes more than 8.9 million fractures annually, which means that on average, an osteoporotic fracture occurs every 3 seconds (1). In this chapter we describe the burden placed on individuals, healthcare systems and societies globally by osteoporotic fractures.

GLOBAL BURDEN OF OSTEOPOROSIS AND FRACTURE

The Global Burden of Disease study demonstrated the massive impact of musculoskeletal conditions on populations worldwide: the number of disability adjusted life years (DALYs) attributable to musculoskeletal disorders has increased by 17.7% between 2005 and 2013 (2). 'Low back pain' ranked top, 'neck pain' fourth, 'other musculoskeletal' tenth and 'osteoarthritis' thirteenth in the

Table 1.1 Impact of osteoporosis-related fractures across Europe

	Hip	Spine	Wrist
Lifetime risk in women (%)	23	29	21
Lifetime risk in men (%)	11	14	5
Cases/year	620,000	810,000	574,000
Hospitalisation (%)	100	2–10	5
Relative survival	0.83	0.82	1.00

Source: Data derived from Hernlund E et al. Arch Osteoporos. 2013 Dec;8(1-2):136.
Note: Costs: All sites combined ~ €37 billion.

WHO rankings of causes for years lived with disability worldwide in 2013 (3), with osteoporotic fractures playing a major part in the 'back pain' and 'other musculoskeletal' categories. The 2004 US Surgeon General's report estimated that 10 million Americans over the age of 50 years have osteoporosis, leading to 1.5 million fragility fractures of the hip, spine, wrist, humerus, pelvis, scapula or ribs each year (4), with another 34 million Americans at risk of the disease. The cost to the US is around $17.9 billion per annum. Currently the US National Osteoporosis Foundation estimates that 54 million Americans suffer from either osteoporosis or osteopenia (5). In the European Union (EU), a report estimated that in 2010, 6.6% of men and 22.1% of women aged over 50 years had osteoporosis, and that there were 3.5 million fragility fractures (6). The annual direct costs attributable to fracture treatment in the EU equate to approximately €24 billion, though when indirect costs such as long-term care and fracture prevention therapies are taken into account, this figure rises to €37 billion per year across the 27 countries of the EU (6) Table 1.1. This amounted to 1,180,000 quality-adjusted life-years lost during 2010.

A British study indicated similar population risks (7), with 1 in 2 women and 1 in 5 men aged 50 years expected to have an osteoporosis-related fracture in their remaining lifetime. In addition to the associated morbidity and economic cost, fractures are associated with an increased mortality, with hip fractures associated with an excess mortality of 10% to 20% in the first year after fracture (8), with a similar proportion requiring long-term residential or nursing care (9,10).

Owing to the ageing population, global costs of osteoporotic fracture are expected to increase by 25% during the period 2010–2025 (6). A similar increase is predicted in the United States, where osteoporosis is the 10th ranked major illness and is among the top 5% highest cost Medicare beneficiaries (4).

VARIATION IN FRACTURE RATES BY AGE AND SEX

Fracture incidence in the community is bimodal, showing peaks in youth and in the very elderly (11,12). In young people, fractures of long bones predominate, often after substantial trauma, and are more frequent in males than females. For example, rates of skull, carpus, clavicle, ankle and lower leg fracture, all classically associated with high trauma such as road traffic accidents, are particularly frequent in young males; in contrast, hip fractures are uncommon at young ages in both sexes (11,12). In this group the question of bone strength rarely arises, although there are now data suggesting that this may not be entirely irrelevant as a risk factor (13). This distribution is demonstrated in Figure 1.1, from a recent UK study using General Practice (GP) records (the Clinical Practice Research Datalink, CPRD). Over the age of 50 years, fracture incidence in women begins to climb steeply, and rates become twice those in men; note the difference in *y*-axis scales in Figure 1.1. It is also important to note that rates of vertebral fracture are underestimated when relying on clinical diagnosis alone – vertebral fracture, when ascertained from radiographs rather than clinical presentation, makes a significant contribution to fracture rates, as shown in Figure 1.2 (14).

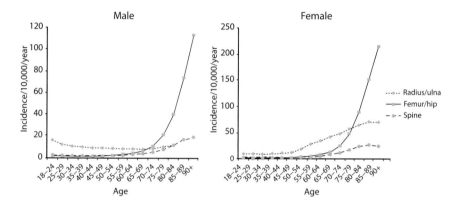

Figure 1.1 Age- and sex-specific rates of fracture at the radius/ulna, femur/hip and spine, from the UK CPRD, 1988–2012. (Reproduced with permission from Curtis EM et al. *Bone.* 2016;87:19-26.)

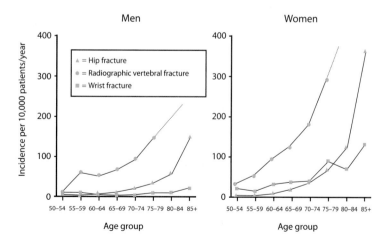

Figure 1.2 Radiographic vertebral, and hip and wrist fracture incidence by age and sex. (Adapted with permission from van Staa TP et al. *Bone.* 2001;29(6):517-22 and Felsenberg D et al. *J Bone Miner Res.* 2002;17(4):716-24.)

EPIDEMIOLOGY OF HIP, SPINE AND WRIST FRACTURES

Hip fracture

Hip fractures increase exponentially with age in most populations, having a female to male incidence ratio of around two to one, with around 98% occurring among people aged 35 years or over, and 80% occurring in women (11). Seasonal variation in hip fractures is seen in temperate countries, with an increase in winter. It could be assumed that slipping on icy pavements could be a cause for this increase; however, the fact that most hip fractures occur indoors means that this seasonal variation may be due to lower light and slowed neuromuscular reflexes in the winter, possibly related to vitamin D status.

Factors such as ethnicity, geographic location and socioeconomic status have all been shown to influence hip fracture incidence (11), even within a country. In terms of variation by ethnicity, in a recent UK study, fracture rates in white individuals aged over 50 years were three to five times greater than in black individuals (Figure 1.3), with the South Asian population and people of mixed ethnicity experiencing an intermediate fracture rate. This finding has been confirmed in other studies from Scotland, Sweden, South Africa and the United States (15,16). In a Californian study of hip fracture rates, fracture rates of 14.1 per 10,000 person years were demonstrated in white women over 50 years of age, 5.7 per 10,000 person years in black women and 8.5 per 10,000 person years in Asian women (16). The underlying reasons for this have been suggested in studies using hip structural analysis and high resolution peripheral quantitative computed tomography (pQCT) scanning; differences in proximal femoral geometry (shorter, wider femoral neck in black than white individuals) and differences in the bone microarchitecture (with larger, denser bones with higher cortical area, thickness and volume in black than white women) (17). Differences in height and body

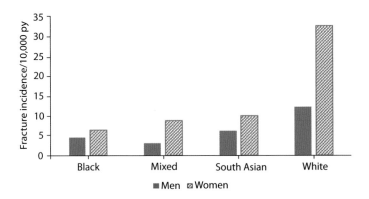

Figure 1.3 Incidence of hip/femur and fragility fractures by ethnicity in men and women aged over 50 years in the UK. (Data from UK Clinical Practice Research Datalink, 1988–2012; adapted with permission from Curtis EM et al. *Bone.* 2016;87:19-26.)

composition between different ethnic groups may also partly explain underlying differences in fracture rates; white individuals are generally taller than Asian and black individuals, as demonstrated by data from the National Health and Nutrition Examination Survey (NHANES) cohort (18). Body height has been shown to have an independent influence on hip fracture rates, with taller individuals at greater risk (19).

Deprivation has also been shown to be associated with hip fractures in particular, and more in men than women in various populations including the UK, US and Netherlands (11,20–22). In the UK CPRD study, the relative risk of hip fracture was 1.3 in index of multiple deprivation category 5 (most deprived), compared to category 1 (see Figure 1.4), possibly due to adverse lifestyle factors with known effects on bone health, such as poor dietary quality, smoking and alcohol use clustering with low socioeconomic status (20–24). The prevalence of obesity is also greater amongst populations of lower, compared with higher, socioeconomic status but this would be expected to have diverging effects on fracture incidence dependent on fracture site. For example, a recent meta-analysis demonstrated that obesity is protective for hip fracture but is associated with increased risk of ankle fracture (25).

There is considerable excess mortality following a hip fracture, with around 31,000 excess deaths within 6 months of the approximately 300,000 hip fractures that occur annually in the US. The risk of death is greatest immediately post-fracture, and decreases gradually over time. About 8% of men and 3% of women aged >50 years die whilst hospitalised for their fracture, and hip fracture is higher in men than women, increases with age and, as would be expected, is greater for those with co-existing illnesses (26). A large meta-analysis showed that mortality in the year post hip fracture ranges from 20% to 26% amongst elderly females and males respectively (27), supported by a UK study which showed 1-year all-cause mortality from hip fracture to be 22.3% in 2000–2008 (26). Reduced survival has been shown to be associated with all types of fracture except for minor fractures (where mortality was increased only for those aged 75 years or older).

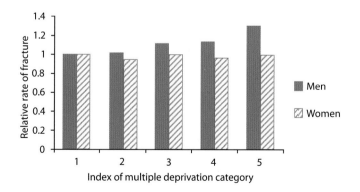

Figure 1.4 Incidence of hip fracture by fifths of socioeconomic deprivation in the UK. (Greater index of Multiple Deprivation Category = more deprivation). (Reproduced with permission from Curtis EM et al. *Bone.* 2016;87:19-26.)

Although mortality risk is at its most elevated in the early post fracture period (5–8 times in the first 3 months following a hip fracture), it has been shown to persist for up to 10 years afterwards (27,28).

Morbidity is also considerable following hip fracture, with patients prone to developing complications such as pneumonia, urinary tract infections and pressure sores. In the long term, the ability to walk independently is reduced to 50% in those individuals who were ambulatory prior to hip fracture (9). Cognitive impairment, comorbidity and age are important determinants of a successful outcome (29), as evidenced by the fact that 14% of 50- to 55-year-old hip fracture sufferers are discharged to nursing homes, versus 55% of those >90 years old (30).

Vertebral fracture

Vertebral fractures (of which the major clinical consequences are back pain, kyphosis and height loss), are more difficult to quantify than hip fractures, mainly because they are often asymptomatic and there are disagreements about the radiographic definitions of vertebral deformities. In studies using radiographic screening of populations, the incidence of vertebral fractures has been estimated to be around three times the incidence of hip fracture, though only around one–third of vertebral fractures come to medical attention (Figure 1.2) (7,14). Data from the European Vertebral Osteoporosis Study (EVOS), which counts radiographically determined vertebral fractures, have shown that the age-standardised population prevalence across Europe was 12.2% for men and 12.0% for women aged 50–79 years (31). However, a recently published systematic review suggested that the rates of radiographically determined vertebral fracture are much higher – with a prevalence rate of 26% in Scandinavian women, 18% in Eastern European women and 20–24% in North American white women aged ≥50, with a white:black ratio of 1.6. Rates in Latin America were in general lower than in Europe and North America, and varied widely throughout Asia and the Middle East (32).

In the past, it was believed that vertebral fractures were more common in men than women. EVOS data, however, suggest that this is only the case at younger ages – here the frequency of vertebral deformities on spinal radiographs is similar in men and women, if not slightly higher in men, probably due to the greater incidence of trauma. At older ages, vertebral fractures are more common in women, with the majority occurring through normal activities such as lifting of non-heavy items, rather than through falling. In EVOS, at age 75–79 years, the incidence of radiologically defined vertebral fractures was 13.6 per 1000 person years for men and 29.3 per 1000 person years for women (14). In contrast, in an earlier study from Rochester, Minnesota, in which vertebral fractures were defined by clinical presentation, the incidence was 0.2 per 1000 person years for men and 9.8 per 1000 person years in 75- to 84-year-olds (33).

Somewhat surprisingly, vertebral fractures are associated with increased mortality well beyond 1 year post-fracture (28,34), with co-morbid conditions contributing significantly to the decreased relative survival. In contrast to hip fractures, where the mortality risk is highest in the time period closest to the fracture, the impairment of survival following a vertebral fracture markedly worsens as time from diagnosis of the fracture increases. In the UK CPRD, the observed survival in women 12 months after vertebral fracture was 86.5% versus 93.6% expected, whilst at 5 years survival was 56.5% observed and 69.9% expected (7). As would be predicted, quality of life (QUALEFFO) scores decrease as the number of vertebral fractures increases (35).

Distal forearm fracture

Wrist fracture rates increase gradually with age, in contrast to the exponential increases in hip fractures at older ages (Figure 1.2) (11). At older ages, rates are higher in women than men, with the incidence 39.7 per 10,000 person years and 8.9 per 10,000 person years, respectively in the UK for individuals aged 50 years or greater (11). Overall, despite impacting on some activities such as writing and meal preparation few patients are completely disabled by wrist fractures, despite over half reporting only fair to poor function at 6 months (30). These fractures do not appear to increase mortality (7).

RISK OF SUBSEQUENT FRACTURE WITHIN INDIVIDUALS

Studies suggest that patients with previous fragility fractures are at risk of subsequent fractures of any type. In a meta-analysis of 15,259 men and 44,902 women across 11 population cohorts, a history of prior fracture was shown to be associated with an 86% increase in the risk of any new fracture (36). In a UK study of over 30,000 hip fracture patients, the risk of subsequent fracture was high; 14.7% suffered a major non-hip fragility fracture (of the vertebrae, humerus or forearm), and 32.5% any fracture, within 5 years of their hip fracture (37). The EVOS study of vertebral fractures demonstrated even higher risks, such that prevalent vertebral deformity predicted incident hip fracture with a rate ratio of 2.8–4.5, and this increased with the number of vertebral deformities present at baseline (38). Although not characterised in detail, there is evidence from a Swedish study that risk of subsequent fracture is particularly high in the period immediately after the index fracture (39), providing a rationale for early intervention with anti-osteoporosis therapies after fracture.

GENETIC INFLUENCES ON FRACTURE RISK

Considering the differences in fracture rates between ethnically different populations, it is important to understand the genetic influences on fracture risk. There appears to be substantial heritability of bone mass, as determined by twin and family studies (40,41). Areal BMD appears to be characterised by high heritability (h^2), estimated to be 45% to 78% depending upon the skeletal site and age (42,43). Initial research focused on several likely candidate genes, including the vitamin D receptor gene (VDR) (44), IL-6 (45), collagen 1α1 (46), TGFβ (47) and LDL receptor-related protein 5 (LRP5) (48). Many genome-wide association studies (GWAS) and their meta-analyses have been conducted for BMD and dozens of genomic loci have been identified, some of which are noncoding variants (e.g. EN1, near the WNT16 gene), and many of which occur with low minor allele frequency (MAF) (49,50). So far, individual loci detected through GWAS studies only explain approximately 5% of the variance in BMD (51), but there is increasing evidence from whole-genome sequencing that low frequency, non-coding variants could explain a proportion of the missing heritability (49,52).

Moreover, it has been shown that in spite of the strong heritable component of aBMD, the genes identified in GWAS so far only overlap to some degree with the fracture phenotype (53). GWAS linked to HRpQCT analyses are now emerging that provide measures of trabecular and cortical traits, which may be more important predictors of fracture (54). Despite the suggestion that further variance will be explained by next-generation sequencing approaches, but there is growing evidence that some of the residual variance might be explained by interaction between genes and environment, both in utero and in early life (55). This may occur for example by epigenetic regulatory processes, which are discussed in Chapter 8.

GLOBAL VARIATION IN FRACTURE RATES

Global variation in fracture incidence is best documented for hip fracture, and studies have shown marked heterogeneity in annual age-standardised hip fracture rates. The largest systematic review, published in 2012, used a literature survey covering a 50-year period and UN data on population demography (56). The highest annual age-standardised hip fracture incidences (per 100,000 person years) were observed in Scandinavia (Denmark [574], Norway [563] and Sweden [539], plus Austria [501]). The lowest were found in Nigeria [2], South Africa [20], Tunisia [57] and Ecuador [58]. In general, there was a swathe of high-risk countries in Northwestern Europe, Central Europe, the Russian Federation and Middle-Eastern countries such as Iran, Kuwait and Oman. Other high-risk countries were Hong Kong, Singapore and Taiwan. Generally low-risk regions included Latin America (with the exception of Argentina), Africa and Saudi Arabia, as shown in Figure 1.5. There was around a tenfold range in hip fracture incidence worldwide, with the overall age-standardised incidence in men being half that of women. The highest incidence of hip fractures was generally observed in countries furthest from the equator and in countries in which extensive coverage of the skin due to religious or cultural practices is the norm, which suggests that vitamin D status may be an important factor underlying this distribution.

Using the FRAX models (where available), the 10-year probability of major osteoporotic fracture (hip, clinical vertebral, forearm or humeral fracture) was calculated by country for individuals with a BMD at the threshold for a diagnosis of osteoporosis (T score −2.5). As shown in Figure 1.6, in both men and women the lowest probabilities were found in Tunisia, Ecuador, the Philippines and China, with the highest rates in Denmark, Sweden, Norway and Switzerland, with the United States (Caucasian population data only) fifth highest and the UK ninth highest. Fracture probabilities were on average 23% higher in women than men, as opposed to overall hip fracture incidence which was twofold higher in

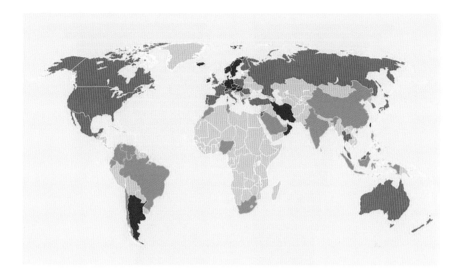

Figure 1.5 Hip fracture rates for men and women combined in different countries of the world categorised by risk, countries are coded red (annual incidence >250/100,000), orange (150–250/100,000) or green (<150/100,000) where estimates are available. (Reproduced with permission from Kanis JA et al. *Osteoporos Int.* 2012;23(9):2239-56.)

women than in men. This closer approximation between the sexes for the probability estimate (which included a BMD measurement) arises because the risk of hip and other osteoporotic fracture is roughly identical in men and women of the same age and femoral neck BMD (57–59). The slightly higher probability estimate seen in women reflects the lower death risk in women compared with men.

The reasons for such large worldwide variation in age- and sex-adjusted hip fracture incidence are not clear. Some of the differences may be attributed to systematic errors and bias; clearly, inaccurate coding and recording of fractures may occur between countries; some countries used regional estimates which may not be representative of overall fracture risk, and the studies were performed over a long period – over 20% of the included studies were conducted more than a decade previously. Additionally, in some areas of the world, not all hip fracture cases come to medical attention [e.g. in Georgia, Kazakhstan and Kyrgyzstan over 50% are not hospitalised (60) due to poor access to surgical services and affordable medical care]. However, such problems would not undermine the principal finding of tenfold differences in hip fracture risk, and in 10-year fracture probability worldwide. Genetic differences in bone structure according to ethnicity may go some way towards explaining the differences in fracture risk, but the fact that immigrant populations show acclimatisation to local fracture rates (for example, the incidence of hip fracture in black North Americans is much higher than in black African populations) (61), suggests that environmental factors are more important (62). Socioeconomic prosperity is thought to be an important factor leading to lower levels of physical activity

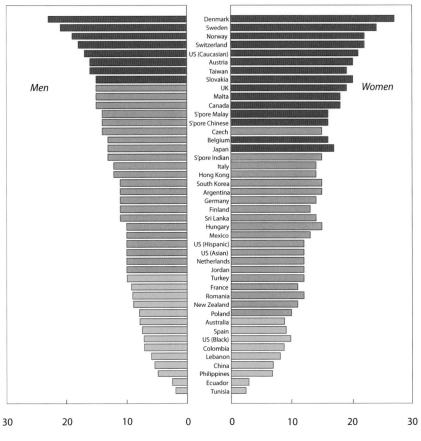

30   20   10   0   0   10   20   30

10 year probability (%)

Figure 1.6 Ten-year probability of major fracture (in percent) in men and women aged 65 years with a prior fragility fracture and no other clinical risk factors, with a BMI of 24 kg/m² at the threshold of osteoporosis as judged by BMD at the femoral neck (i.e. T-score −2.5). Probability in different countries is categorised as high (red, >15%), moderate (orange, 10–15%) and low (green, <10%). (Reproduced with permission from Kanis JA et al. *Osteoporos Int.* 2012;23(9):2239-56.)

and the increased probability of falling onto hard surfaces (indeed a US$10,000 higher GDP per capita was associated with a 1.3% increase in hip fracture probability) (63). However, within countries, higher socioeconomic status appears to have a protective effect against hip fractures in both the US and UK (11,20). Calcium intake is another example of a risk factor, whereby its role as a risk factor within populations (low calcium intake being an independent risk factor for osteoporosis) (64) appears to have opposite associations when countries are compared (high nutritional calcium intake countries having greater hip fracture risks) (65,66). It is not yet clear which factors overall are causally related to the worldwide heterogeneity in fracture risk.

GLOBAL TRENDS IN FRACTURE INCIDENCE OVER TIME AND FUTURE PROJECTIONS

Current estimates suggest that 12% of the world population (around 901 million people) are over the age of 60 years. Europe has the greatest percentage of its population aged 60+ years (24%); however, rapid ageing of the population is also occurring in other parts of the world – by the year 2050 all continents except Africa will have nearly a quarter or more of their populations aged 60+ years. The number of older people in the world is projected to be 1.4 billion by 2030 and 2.1 billion by 2050, and could rise to 3.2 billion by 2100 (67).

This growth in the world population and the increasing proportions of older people will substantially impact the number of hip fractures globally in coming decades, with a conservative estimate of the annual number of hip fractures increasing from 1.66 million in 1990 to 6.26 million in 2050, with the latter figure potentially over 20 million when known secular trends are considered (68,69). Trends in age- and sex-adjusted incidence rates have been documented most robustly for hip fracture (Figure 1.7), with studies showing a positive annual change to the right, and negative to the left (70). In many developed countries, age- and sex-specific hip fracture rates appeared to have plateaued or decreased in the last one to two decades, following a rise in preceding years; however in many areas of the developing world, rates are still rising (70).

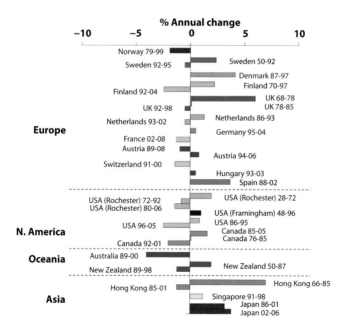

Figure 1.7 Trends in hip fracture worldwide over time: annual change in age and sex-adjusted hip fracture incidence. (Reproduced with permission from Cooper C et al. *Osteoporos Int.* 2011;22(5):1277-88.)

A recent study of UK fracture incidence showed little change in fracture incidence overall from 1990 to 2012, though a small increase in male hip fracture rates was seen (10.8 to 13.4 per 10,000 person-years) (71). In Asia, secular trends in hip fracture rates are heterogeneous – rates in Hong Kong, China appeared to have stabilised between 1985 and 1995 following a steep increase in incidence up to this point (72). Conversely, rates in Beijing have increased by around 33% between 1988 and 1992 from being among the lowest in the world, though this may be due to improvements in the completeness and accuracy of reporting in hospitals (73). In Singapore, one of the most urbanised parts of Asia, hip fracture incidence appeared to be increasing by around 1% per year between 1991 and 1998 in comparison with rates derived from 1965 (74). In Japan, ongoing age- and sex-specific increases in hip fracture rates of around 3.8% per year were recorded in 2006, and a 32% increase in age- and sex-standardised fracture rates was observed between the periods 1992 to 1994 and 2010 to 2012 (75). Such increases, as seen in Singapore, Japan and Hong Kong, appear to be in line with rapid increases in urbanisation, with consequent changes in physical activity and nutrition.

In addition to assessment of the burden of osteoporosis in terms of consequent fracture, there is value in identifying the number of individuals at high fracture risk to help to inform future health resource allocation. Using this approach, it has been estimated that worldwide in 2010 there were 21 million men and 137 million women aged 50 years or greater at high fracture risk, and that this number is expected to double by 2040, with the increase predominantly borne by Asia, Africa and Latin America (76), demonstrated in Figure 1.8. Such increases in the burden of osteoporosis across the world highlight the need for an awareness of the problem facing many populations, and effective primary and secondary prevention strategies for osteoporotic fracture.

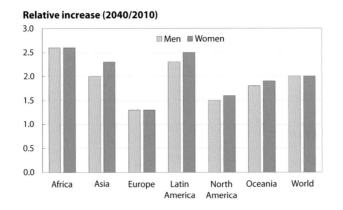

Figure 1.8 Number of men and women at high fracture risk in 2040 relative to 2010, by world region. (Reproduced with permission from Oden A et al. *Osteoporos Int.* 2015;26(9):2243-8.)

CONCLUSION

It is clear that osteoporosis presents a major public health burden, given its high prevalence and associated fragility fractures. There is significant variation in fracture rates by age and sex, with older people at much greater risk than younger people and rates higher in women than men, particularly from the time of the menopause. Substantial geographic variation has been noted in the incidence of osteoporotic fractures worldwide, with Western populations (North America, Europe and Oceania) reporting increases in hip fracture throughout the second half of the twentieth century, with a stabilisation or decline in the last two decades. In developing populations however, particularly in Asia, the rates of osteoporotic fracture appear to be increasing. The massive global burden consequent to osteoporosis means that fracture risk assessment should be a high priority amongst health measures considered by policy makers.

REFERENCES

1. Johnell O, Kanis JA. An estimate of the worldwide prevalence and disability associated with osteoporotic fractaures. *Osteoporos Int.* 2006;17(12):1726-33.

2. Murray CJ, Barber RM, Foreman KJ, Abbasoglu Ozgoren A, Abd-Allah F, Abera SF, et al. Global, regional, and national disability-adjusted life years (DALYs) for 306 diseases and injuries and healthy life expectancy (HALE) for 188 countries, 1990-2013: Quantifying the epidemiological transition. *Lancet.* 2015 Nov 28;386(10009):2145-91. PubMed PMID: 26321261. PubMed Central PMCID: PMC4673910. Epub 2015/09/01. eng.

3. Global, regional, and national incidence, prevalence, and years lived with disability for 301 acute and chronic diseases and injuries in 188 countries, 1990-2013: A systematic analysis for the Global Burden of Disease Study 2013. *Lancet.* 2015 Aug 22;386(9995): 743-800. PubMed PMID: 26063472. PubMed Central PMCID: PMC4561509. Epub 2015/06/13. eng.

4. Office of the Surgeon General (US). Bone Health and Osteoporosis: A Report of the Surgeon General. Rockville MD; 2004.

5. National Osteoporosis Foundation. Annual Report 2015. https://cdnno forg/wp-content/uploads/2017/03/Annual-Report-2015pdf. 2015.

6. Hernlund E, Svedbom A, Ivergard M, Compston J, Cooper C, Stenmark J, et al. Osteoporosis in the European Union: Medical management, epidemiology and economic burden: A report prepared in collaboration with the International Osteoporosis Foundation (IOF) and the European Federation of Pharmaceutical Industry Associations (EFPIA). *Arch Osteoporos.* 2013 Dec;8(1-2):136. PubMed PMID: 24113837. Epub 2013/10/12. eng.

7. van Staa TP, Dennison EM, Leufkens HG, Cooper C. Epidemiology of fractures in England and Wales. *Bone.* 2001 Dec;29(6):517-22. PubMed PMID: 11728921. Epub 2001/12/01. eng.

8. Center JR, Nguyen TV, Schneider D, Sambrook PN, Eisman JA. Mortality after all major types of osteoporotic fracture in men and women: An observational study. *Lancet*. 1999;353(9156):878-82.

9. Compston J, Cooper A, Cooper C, Francis R, Kanis JA, Marsh D, et al. Guidelines for the diagnosis and management of osteoporosis in post-menopausal women and men from the age of 50 years in the UK. *Maturitas*. 2009;62(2):105-8.

10. Harvey N, Dennison E, Cooper C. Osteoporosis: Impact on health and economics. *Nat Rev Rheumatol*. 2010;6(2):99-105.

11. Curtis EM, van der Velde R, Moon RJ, van den Bergh JP, Geusens P, de Vries F, et al. Epidemiology of fractures in the United Kingdom 1988-2012: Variation with age, sex, geography, ethnicity and socioeconomic status. *Bone*. 2016 Jun;87:19-26. PubMed PMID: 26968752. PubMed Central PMCID: PMC4890652. Epub 2016/03/13. eng.

12. Moon RJ, Harvey NC, Curtis EM, de Vries F, van Staa T, Cooper C. Ethnic and geographic variations in the epidemiology of childhood fractures in the United Kingdom. *Bone*. 2016 Apr;85:9-14. PubMed PMID: 26802259. PubMed Central PMCID: PMC4841386. Epub 2016/01/24. eng.

13. Goulding A, Jones IE, Taylor RW, Manning PJ, Williams SM. More broken bones: A 4-year double cohort study of young girls with and without distal forearm fractures. *J Bone Miner Res*. 8610640. 2000;15(10):2011-8.

14. Felsenberg D, Silman AJ, Lunt M, Armbrecht G, Ismail AA, Finn JD, et al. Incidence of vertebral fracture in Europe: Results from the European Prospective Osteoporosis Study (EPOS). *J Bone Miner Res*. 2002 Apr; 17(4):716-24. PubMed PMID: 11918229. Epub 2002/03/29. eng.

15. Solomon L. Osteoporosis and fracture of the femoral neck in the South African Bantu. *J Bone Joint Surg Br*. 1968 Feb;50(1):2-13. PubMed PMID: 5641595. Epub 1968/02/01. eng.

16. Silverman SL, Madison RE. Decreased incidence of hip fracture in Hispanics, Asians, and blacks: California Hospital Discharge Data. *Am J Public Health*. 1988;78(11):1482-3. PubMed PMID: PMC1350247.

17. Putman MS, Yu EW, Lee H, Neer RM, Schindler E, Taylor AP, et al. Differences in skeletal microarchitecture and strength in African-American and white women. *J Bone Miner Res*. 2013 Oct;28(10):2177-85. PubMed PMID: 23572415. PubMed Central PMCID: Pmc3779478. Epub 2013/04/11. eng.

18. Heymsfield SB, Peterson CM, Thomas DM, Heo M, Schuna JM, Jr., Hong S, et al. Scaling of adult body weight to height across sex and race/ethnic groups: Relevance to BMI. *Am J Clin Nutr*. 2014 Dec;100(6):1455-61. PubMed PMID: 25411280. PubMed Central PMCID: Pmc4232013. Epub 2014/11/21. eng.

19. Meyer HE, Tverdal A, Falch JA. Risk factors for hip fracture in middle-aged Norwegian women and men. *Am J Epidemiol*. 1993 Jun 1;137(11): 1203-11. PubMed PMID: 8322761. Epub 1993/06/01. eng.

20. Bacon WE, Hadden WC. Occurrence of hip fractures and socioeconomic position. *J Aging Health*. 2000;12(2):193-203.

21. Brennan SL, Holloway KL, Williams LJ, Kotowicz MA, Bucki-Smith G, Moloney DJ, et al. The social gradient of fractures at any skeletal site in men and women: Data from the Geelong Osteoporosis Study Fracture Grid. *Osteoporos Int*. 2015;26(4):1351-9.

22. Reyes C, Garcia-Gil M, Elorza JM, Fina-Aviles F, Mendez-Boo L, Hermosilla E, et al. Socioeconomic status and its association with the risk of developing hip fractures: A region-wide ecological study. *Bone*. 2015;73:127-31.

23. Cauley JA, Chalhoub D, Kassem AM, Fuleihan Gel H. Geographic and ethnic disparities in osteoporotic fractures. *Nat Rev Endocrinol*. 2014; 10(6):338-51.

24. Benetou V, Orfanos P, Feskanich D, Michaelsson K, Pettersson-Kymmer U, Eriksson S, et al. Fruit and Vegetable Intake and Hip Fracture Incidence in Older Men and Women: The CHANCES Project. *J Bone Miner Res*. 2016;31(9):1743-52.

25. Johansson H, Kanis JA, Oden A, McCloskey E, Chapurlat RD, Christiansen C, et al. A meta-analysis of the association of fracture risk and body mass index in women. *J Bone Miner Res*. 2014 Jan;29(1):223-33. PubMed PMID: 23775829. Epub 2013/06/19. eng.

26. Klop C, Welsing PM, Cooper C, Harvey NC, Elders PJ, Bijlsma JW, et al. Mortality in British hip fracture patients, 2000-2010: A population-based retrospective cohort study. *Bone*. 2014 Sep;66:171-7. PubMed PMID: 24933345. Epub 2014/06/17. eng.

27. Haentjens P, Magaziner J, Colon-Emeric CS, Vanderschueren D, Milisen K, Velkeniers B, et al. Meta-analysis: Excess mortality after hip fracture among older women and men. *Ann Intern Med*. 2010 Mar 16;152(6):380-90. PubMed PMID: 20231569. PubMed Central PMCID: PMC3010729. Epub 2010/03/17. eng.

28. Bliuc D, Nguyen ND, Milch VE, Nguyen TV, Eisman JA, Center JR. Mortality risk associated with low-trauma osteoporotic fracture and subsequent fracture in men and women. *JAMA*. 2009;301(5):513-21.

29. Kim S-M, Moon Y-W, Lim S-J, Yoon B-K, Min Y-K, Lee D-Y, et al. Prediction of survival, second fracture, and functional recovery following the first hip fracture surgery in elderly patients. *Bone*. 2012 Jun;50(6):1343-50.

30. Chrischilles EA, Butler CD, Davis CS, Wallace RB. A model of lifetime osteoporosis impact. *Arch Intern Med*. 1991 Oct;151(10):2026-32. PubMed PMID: 1929691. Epub 1991/10/01. eng.

31. O'Neill TW, Felsenberg D, Varlow J, Cooper C, Kanis JA, Silman AJ. The prevalence of vertebral deformity in european men and women: The European Vertebral Osteoporosis Study. *J Bone Miner Res*. 1996;11(7):1010-8.

32. Ballane G, Cauley JA, Luckey MM, El-Hajj Fuleihan G. Worldwide preva-
    lence and incidence of osteoporotic vertebral fractures. *Osteoporos Int.*
    2017 May;28(5):1531-42. PubMed PMID: 28168409. Epub 2017/02/09. eng.

33. Cooper C, Atkinson EJ, O'Fallon WM, Melton LJ. Incidence of clinically
    diagnosed vertebral fractures: A population-based study in Rochester,
    Minnesota, 1985-1989. *J Bone Miner Res.* 1992;7(2):221-7.

34. Cooper C, Atkinson EJ, Jacobsen SJ, O'Fallon WM, Melton LJ.
    Population-based study of survival after osteoporotic fractures. *Am J
    Epidemiol.* 1993;137(9):1001-5.

35. Oleksik A, Lips P, Dawson A, Minshall ME, Shen W, Cooper C, et al.
    Health-related quality of life in postmenopausal women with low BMD
    with or without prevalent vertebral fractures [In Process Citation]. *J Bone
    Miner Res.* 2000;15(7):1384-92.

36. Kanis JA, Johnell O, De Laet C, Johansson H, Oden A, Delmas P, et al.
    A meta-analysis of previous fracture and subsequent fracture risk. *Bone.*
    2004 Aug;35(2):375-82. PubMed PMID: 15268886. Epub 2004/07/23. eng.

37. Gibson-Smith D, Klop C, Elders PJ, Welsing PM, van Schoor N, Leufkens
    HG, et al. The risk of major and any (non-hip) fragility fracture after hip
    fracture in the United Kingdom: 2000-2010. *Osteoporos Int.* 2014 Nov;
    25(11):2555-63. PubMed PMID: 25001987. Epub 2014/07/09. eng.

38. Ismail AA, Cockerill W, Cooper C, Finn JD, Abendroth K, Parisi G, et al.
    Prevalent vertebral deformity predicts incident hip though not distal
    forearm fracture: Results from the European Prospective Osteoporosis
    Study. *Osteoporos Int.* 2001;12(2):85-90.

39. Johnell O, Kanis JA, Oden A, Sernbo I, Redlund-Johnell I, Petterson C,
    et al. Fracture risk following an osteoporotic fracture. *Osteoporos Int.*
    2004 Mar;15(3):175-9. PubMed PMID: 14691617. Epub 2003/12/24. eng.

40. Pocock NA, Eisman JA, Hopper JL, Yeates MG, Sambrook PN, Eberl S.
    Genetic determinants of bone mass in adults. A twin study. *J Clin Invest.*
    1987 Sep;80(3):706-10. PubMed PMID: 3624485. PubMed Central PMCID:
    Pmc442294. Epub 1987/09/01. eng.

41. Videman T, Levalahti E, Battie MC, Simonen R, Vanninen E, Kaprio J.
    Heritability of BMD of femoral neck and lumbar spine: A multivariate
    twin study of Finnish men. *J Bone Miner Res.* 2007 Sep;22(9):1455-62.
    PubMed PMID: 17547536. Epub 2007/06/06. eng.

42. Liu C-T, Karasik D, Zhou Y, Hsu Y-H, Genant HK, Broe KE, et al. Heritability
    of prevalent vertebral fracture and volumetric bone mineral density and
    geometry at the lumbar spine in three generations of the framingham
    study. *J Bone Miner Res.* 2012;27(4):954-8.

43. Ralston SH, de Crombrugghe B. Genetic regulation of bone mass and
    susceptibility to osteoporosis. *Genes Devel.* 2006 September 15, 2006;
    20(18):2492-506.

44. Langdahl BL, Gravholt CH, Brixen K, Eriksen EF. Polymorphisms in the
    vitamin D receptor gene and bone mass, bone turnover and osteoporotic
    fractures [see comments]. *Eur J Clin Invest.* 2000;30(7):608-17.

45. Nordstrom A, Gerdhem P, Brandstrom H, Stiger F, Lerner UH, Lorentzon M, et al. Interleukin-6 promoter polymorphism is associated with bone quality assessed by calcaneus ultrasound and previous fractures in a cohort of 75-year-old women. *Osteoporos Int.* 2004;15(10):820-6.

46. Mann V, Hobson EE, Li B, Stewart TL, Grant SF, Robins SP, et al. A COL1A1 Sp1 binding site polymorphism predisposes to osteoporotic fracture by affecting bone density and quality. *J Clin Invest.* 2001;107(7):899-907.

47. Hinke V, Seck T, Clanget C, Scheidt-Nave C, Ziegler R, Pfeilschifter J. Association of transforming growth factor-beta1 (TGFbeta1) T29 —> C gene polymorphism with bone mineral density (BMD), changes in BMD, and serum concentrations of TGF-beta1 in a population-based sample of post-menopausal german women. *Calcif Tissue Int.* 2001;69(6):315-20.

48. Koay MA, Tobias JH, Leary SD, Steer CD, Vilarino-Guell C, Brown MA. The effect of LRP5 polymorphisms on bone mineral density is apparent in childhood. *Calcif Tissue Int.* 2007;81(1):1-9.

49. Zheng HF, Forgetta V, Hsu YH, Estrada K, Rosello-Diez A, Leo PJ, et al. Whole-genome sequencing identifies EN1 as a determinant of bone density and fracture. *Nature.* 2015 Oct 1;526(7571):112-7. PubMed PMID: 26367794. PubMed Central PMCID: PMC4755714. Epub 2015/09/15. eng.

50. Moayyeri A, Hsu Y-H, Karasik D, Estrada K, Xiao S-M, Nielson C, et al. Genetic determinants of heel bone properties: Genome-wide association meta-analysis and replication in the GEFOS/GENOMOS consortium. *Hum Molec Genet.* 2014 Jun1:23(11):3054-68. Epub 2014/01/14.

51. Richards JB, Zheng HF, Spector TD. Genetics of osteoporosis from genome-wide association studies: Advances and challenges. *Nat Rev Genet.* 2012 Jul 18;13(8):576-88. PubMed PMID: 22805710. Epub 2012/07/19. eng.

52. Yang J, Bakshi A, Zhu Z, Hemani G, Vinkhuyzen AA, Lee SH, et al. Genetic variance estimation with imputed variants finds negligible missing heritability for human height and body mass index. *Nat Genet.* 2015 Oct;47(10):1114-20. PubMed PMID: 26323059. PubMed Central PMCID: PMC4589513. Epub 2015/09/01. eng.

53. Estrada K, Styrkarsdottir U, Evangelou E, Hsu YH, Duncan EL, Ntzani EE, et al. Genome-wide meta-analysis identifies 56 bone mineral density loci and reveals 14 loci associated with risk of fracture. *Nat Genet.* 2012;44(5):491-501.

54. Karasik D, Demissie S, Zhou Y, Lu D, Broe KE, Bouxsein ML, et al. Heritability and Genetic Correlations for Bone Microarchitecture: The Framingham Study Families. *J Bone Miner Res.* 2017 Jan;32(1):106-14. PubMed PMID: 27419666. PubMed Central PMCID: PMC5310688. Epub 2016/10/27. eng.

55. Dennison EM, Arden NK, Keen RW, Syddall H, Day IN, Spector TD, et al. Birthweight, vitamin D receptor genotype and the programming of osteoporosis. *Paediatr Perinat Epidemiol.* 2001;15(3):211-9.

56. Kanis JA, Oden A, McCloskey EV, Johansson H, Wahl DA, Cooper C. A systematic review of hip fracture incidence and probability of fracture worldwide. *Osteoporos Int.* 2012 Sep;23(9):2239-56. PubMed PMID: 22419370. PubMed Central PMCID: PMC3421108. Epub 2012/03/16. eng.

57. Srinivasan B, Kopperdahl DL, Amin S, Atkinson EJ, Camp J, Robb RA, et al. Relationship of femoral neck areal bone mineral density to volumetric bone mineral density, bone size, and femoral strength in men and women. *Osteoporos Int.* 2012;23(1):155-62.

58. Kanis JA, Bianchi G, Bilezikian JP, Kaufman JM, Khosla S, Orwoll E, et al. Towards a diagnostic and therapeutic consensus in male osteoporosis. *Osteoporos Int.* 2011 Nov;22(11):2789-98. PubMed PMID: 21509585. PubMed Central PMCID: PMC3555694. Epub 2011/04/22. eng.

59. Johnell O, Kanis JA, Oden A, Johansson H, De Laet C, Delmas P, et al. Predictive value of BMD for hip and other fractures. *J Bone Miner Res.* 2005;20(7):1185-94.

60. The Eastern European & Central Asian Regional Audit Epidemiology, costs & burden of osteoporosis in 2010. Nyon, Switzerland: International Osteoporosis Foundation, 2011.

61. Cauley JA, El-Hajj Fuleihan G, Arabi A, Fujiwara S, Ragi-Eis S, Calderon A, et al. Official Positions for FRAX(R) clinical regarding international differences from Joint Official Positions Development Conference of the International Society for Clinical Densitometry and International Osteoporosis Foundation on FRAX(R). *J Clin Densitom.* 2011 Jul-Sep;14(3):240-62. PubMed PMID: 21810532. Epub 2011/08/04. eng.

62. Elffors I, Allander E, Kanis JA, Gullberg B, Johnell O, Dequeker J, et al. The variable incidence of hip fracture in southern Europe: The MEDOS Study. *Osteoporos Int.* 1994 Sep;4(5):253-63. PubMed PMID: 7812073. Epub 1994/09/01. eng.

63. Johnell O, Borgstrom F, Jonsson B, Kanis J. Latitude, socioeconomic prosperity, mobile phones and hip fracture risk. *Osteoporos Int.* 2007 Mar;18(3):333-7. PubMed PMID: 17077942. Epub 2006/11/02. eng.

64. Johnell O, Gullberg B, Kanis JA, Allander E, Elffors L, Dequeker J, et al. Risk factors for hip fracture in European women: The MEDOS Study. Mediterranean Osteoporosis Study. *J Bone Miner Res.* 1995;10 (11):1802-15.

65. Kanis JA, Passmore R. Calcium supplementation of the diet – I. *BMJ.* 1989 Jan 21;298(6667):137-40. PubMed PMID: 2493832. PubMed Central PMCID: PMC1835487. Epub 1989/01/21. eng.

66. Kanis JA, Passmore R. Calcium supplementation of the diet – II. *BMJ.* 1989 Jan 28;298(6668):205-8. PubMed PMID: 2493864. PubMed Central PMCID: PMC1835554. Epub 1989/01/28. eng.

67. United Nations. World Population Prospects: 2015 Revision. New York: United Nations, 2015.

68. Cooper C, Campion G, Melton LJ. Hip fractures in the elderly: A worldwide projection. *Osteoporos Int.* 1992;2(6):285-9.

69. Gullberg B, Johnell O, Kanis JA. World-wide projections for hip fracture. *Osteoporos Int.* 1997;7(5):407-13. PubMed PMID: 9425497. Epub 1997 /01/01. eng.

70. Cooper C, Cole ZA, Holroyd CR, Earl SC, Harvey NC, Dennison EM, et al. Secular trends in the incidence of hip and other osteoporotic fractures. *Osteoporos Int.* 2011;22(5):1277-88.

71. van der Velde RY, Wyers CE, Curtis EM, Geusens PP, van den Bergh JP, de Vries F, et al. Secular trends in fracture incidence in the UK between 1990 and 2012. *Osteoporos Int.* 2016 Jun 9. PubMed PMID: 27283403. Epub 2016/06/11. eng.

72. Lau EM, Cooper C, Fung H, Lam D, Tsang KK. Hip fracture in Hong Kong over the last decade – A comparison with the UK. *J Public Health Med.* 1999;21(3):249-50.

73. Xu L, Lu A, Zhao X, Chen X, Cummings SR. Very low rates of hip fracture in Beijing, People's Republic of China the Beijing Osteoporosis Project. *Am J Epidemiol.* 1996;144(9):901-7.

74. Koh LK, Saw SM, Lee JJ, Leong KH, Lee J. Hip fracture incidence rates in Singapore 1991-1998. *Osteoporos Int.* 2001;12(4):311-8. PubMed PMID: 11420781. Epub 2001/06/26. eng.

75. Tsukutani Y, Hagino H, Ito Y, Nagashima H. Epidemiology of fragility fractures in Sakaiminato, Japan: Incidence, secular trends, and prognosis. *Osteoporos Int.* 2015 Sep;26(9):2249-55. PubMed PMID: 25986382. Epub 2015/05/20. eng.

76. Oden A, McCloskey EV, Kanis JA, Harvey NC, Johansson H. Burden of high fracture probability worldwide: Secular increases 2010-2040. *Osteoporos Int.* 2015 Sep;26(9):2243-8. PubMed PMID: 26018089. Epub 2015/05/29. eng.

2

DOHaD: The concept, its implications and applications

MARK HANSON AND CYRUS COOPER

INTRODUCTION

The field of developmental origins of health and disease (DOHaD) is now well established, with a journal (1), an International Society (2) and many hundreds of researchers in over 50 countries engaged in research in this field. The conceptual basis of DOHaD has been the subject of several recent reviews (3–6) and has now been integrated with a range of other disciplines including evolutionary biology (7,8), evo devo (9), anthropology (10), the social sciences (11); and see Chapter 14 in this volume). The field has moved from the epidemiology which described the association between early life and later risk of noncommunicable diseases (12) through a range of studies in animals, which have addressed the mechanistic basis (13,14), to prospective cohort and intervention studies (e.g. 15–18). Rather than rehearsing these issues, in this chapter we focus on the insights DOHaD thinking has given in these three areas.

GLOBAL CHALLENGE OF NONCOMMUNICABLE DISEASES: THE LIFECOURSE MODEL

It is now recognised that noncommunicable diseases (NCDs) account for nearly two-thirds of deaths globally (19) and that their prevalence is increasing, especially in low-middle income countries undergoing economic transitions, and with urbanisation and the adoption of westernised diets and sedentary lifestyle more generally (20). NCDs have been the subject of a United Nations landmark initiative (21). The major NCDs linked with premature mortality are usually considered to be cardiovascular and lung disease, type 2 diabetes and some forms of cancer. Their potential economic impact is large, and although not featured in the Millennium Development Goals, addressing them is a clear target in the Sustainable Development Goals (22). In this context it is important to recognise that many other categories of chronic illness, whilst not necessarily leading directly to death, are nonetheless associated with loss of DALYs and substantial economic costs. Mental illness would come under this category, as would musculoskeletal disorders including the subject of this volume, osteoporosis.

Diseases such as osteoporosis have often been considered an inevitable consequence of the hormonal changes associated with ageing, compounded by poor diet or other unhealthy lifestyle factors, inadequate physical activity, sarcopenia and frailty. Thus they would be expected to be more prevalent as a result of increases in longevity and the demographic shift to a greater proportion of older members of the population, especially in high income countries. More recently, however, there has been recognition that the aetiology of NCDs extends across the lifecourse. This is particularly apparent for risk factors such as obesity. The problem of obesity in increasing risk of NCDs has developed too rapidly to be explicable in purely fixed genetic terms. In addition, adult lifestyle interventions seem to be relatively ineffective (see [23,24] for reviews). Even more alarming is the rise in the prevalence of obesity even in young children. For example in the UK over 33% of boys and girls aged 2–15 years are overweight or obese; for girls and young women this rises to 36% by age 16–24 years and to 50% by age 25–34 years (25). Globally, it is predicted that by 2025 more than 21% of the women in the world will be obese (26).

Such considerations have led to the widespread adoption of a lifecourse model of NCD risk (Figure 2.1). This stresses that primary prevention strategies have to commence early in the lifecourse, even during fetal and infant periods for any generation. Realistically, because the time of conception is often uncertain, about 50% of pregnancies are unplanned, and research has shown that aspects of maternal (and paternal) behaviours – obesity, diet, and characteristics such as maternal age – can effect early embryonic development and also pregnancy outcomes, primordial prevention needs to commence in the preconception period (27). That the nonlinear trajectory of NCDs such as diabetes commences in early life is confirmed by data from both high income and low to middle income countries. A good example are the recent data on hypertension (28). Another is the different lifecourse trajectory of mortality from cardiovascular disease in individuals whose mothers were obese before and in early pregnancy (29). Such a distribution

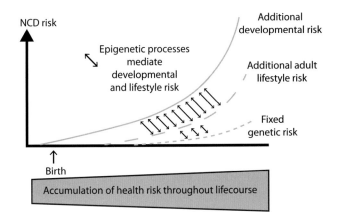

Figure 2.1 The lifecourse model of noncommunicable disease risk, showing its nonlinear trajectory, with a small genetic component amplified by components from unhealthy adult lifestyles, but amplified still more by processes operating during early development starting before birth. Epigenetic processes are thought to underlie many of these processes and their interactions. (Modified with permission from Hanson MA, Godfrey KM. *Nat Rev Endocrinol.* 2015 May 1;11(5):261-3.)

often means that there are many more individuals with higher NCD risk or who are not recognised in primary healthcare than there are known cases. This is true through adolescence and into young adulthood, and because the first contact with a healthcare professional for some women may not be until early pregnancy, especially those in lower socio-economic and educational groups, the opportunity for a truly primordial preventive intervention may have been missed.

FOCUS ON THE PRE-CONCEPTIONAL PHASES OF THE LIFECOURSE

For the reasons above there is now widespread appreciation that the preconception period of the lifecourse may offer a critical opportunity for intervention. This is particularly true of adolescence. The Global Strategy for Women's, Children's and Adolescent's Health states (30):

> Adolescence is a second critical developmental stage. The physical, mental and social potential acquired in childhood can blossom into skills, behaviours and opportunities that contribute to better health and well-being in adolescence and later to a more productive adulthood. The right investments and opportunities may consolidate early gains, or offer a second chance to young people who missed out during childhood. Moreover, as possible future parents, adolescents can transfer health potentials and risks to future generations.

Although the preconception period is arguably quite broad, effectively comprising the reproductive years of women, there are several reasons why a focus on the early part of this period, especially adolescence, is being made. From a demographic perspective, adolescents form an increasing component of the population, especially in low to middle income countries. The Lancet commission on adolescents (31) states 'there are 1.2 billion adolescents in the world today, almost 90% of whom live in developing countries … In many parts of the world, including in high income countries, the lives and prospects of adolescents and young people have deteriorated in recent years'. The latter point is important because this section of the population have received less attention and investment in health than have other groups, for example younger children. This in turn highlights a conceptual problem which has wider implications. The United Nation's Convention on the Rights of the Child (32) is supported by all UN member states with the exception of the United States. It has been followed by a series of comments, of which Comment 4 (33) states that 'adolescents are in general a healthy population group'. This is no longer accurate when viewed from the life-course perspective, because although many adolescents may believe that they are healthy, and indeed may appear outwardly to be so, nonetheless they can be on a high trajectory of risk of later NCDs. A good example of this comes from the study of Twig et al. (34) who showed that the entire range of BMI in adolescents, from underweight to obesity, was related to the risk of death from cardiovascular disease up to 45 years later.

The Global Strategy for Women's, Children's and Adolescents' Health (30) notes a 'ten-fold return on investments in the health and nutrition of women, children and adolescents through later educational attainment, workforce participation and social contributions'. This figure greatly exceeds other returns and emphasises the fundamental importance health across generations plays in the economy of all countries (35). Building on this through greater attention to healthcare, education and social support during childhood also produces very substantial effects across a range of aspects of society (36). The problem is particularly acute in low-middle income countries: it has recently been estimated that 43% of children under 5 years of age in these countries will not achieve their developmental potential, and that this will result in a loss of income in these counties at least twice as large as the proportion of GDP spent on health care (37).

In April 2016 the United Nations General Assembly proclaimed a decade of action on nutrition from 2016 to 2025 (38), calling on governments to 'exercise their primary role and responsibility for addressing undernourishment, stunting, wasting, underweight and overweight in children under 5 years of age, anaemia in women and children – among other micronutrient deficiencies. It also commits them to reverse the rising trends in overweight and obesity and reduce the burden of diet-related non-communicable diseases in all age groups. This complements and enhances the targets set out in the Sustainable Development Goals also launched in late 2015, in particular Goal 2.2 ('By 2030, end all forms of malnutrition, including achieving, by 2025, the internationally agreed targets on stunting and wasting in children under 5 years of age, and address the nutritional needs of adolescent girls, pregnant and lactating women and older persons') and Goal 3.4 ('By 2030, reduce by one third premature mortality from non-communicable diseases through prevention and treatment and promote mental health and well-being').

The lifecourse approach forms a key part of the final report of the WHO Commission on Ending Childhood Obesity (ECHO; 39) published in January 2016, followed by an implementation plan disseminated in January 2017 (40). International professional organisations have similarly focussed on this period of the lifecourse, e.g. the FIGO Adolescent, Preconception and Maternal Nutrition recommendations which emphasise the importance of preventing malnutrition (i.e. both under- and overnutrition) during these periods under the banner of 'Think Nutrition First' (41). Quality rather than quantity of nutrition is emphasised, part of the global agenda of prioritising balanced nutrition for everyone, as is the importance of improving nutritional education in adolescent girls and young women.

RELEVANCE TO THE EARLY ORIGINS OF OSTEOPOROSIS

There has now been considerable work conducted on the early origins of the risk of osteoporosis; much of this is summarised elsewhere in this volume. As with other NCDs, the early research in this area focused on the link with low birthweight and increased later risk (42). Indeed a component of the genetic contribution to the level of bone density or mineral content, e.g. in terms of vitamin D receptor genotype (43), may also be shown to interact with birthweight. Since then, effects of maternal vitamin D status, smoking, level of physical activity and diet during pregnancy on bone mass in young children have all been shown (44). The effects appear to involve epigenetic changes in genes which have functional plausibility in terms of bone development (see Chapters 7 and 8, this volume). Whether these indeed lie on a causal pathway or represent related developmental effects is currently not known. Nonetheless they may serve as valuable biomarkers of later risk which could be used to stratify the population in this respect, to encourage lifestyle modifications such as in diet or physical activity, and to monitor the efficacy of early life interventions to reduce later risk at the population level. Epigenetic marks measured at birth are likely to give a more accurate measure of the foregoing developmental environment than does birthweight, although, as with other research on the links between developmental epigenetics and later risk of NCDs, the issues of whether the marks are sustained, tissue specific or reversible, have not yet been addressed.

The lifecourse model offers a powerful insight into the importance of a developmental approach to chronic disease prevention. The trajectories of bone and skeletal muscle accrual are affected by early development, from fetal life through childhood and adolescence (45). This therefore influences peak bone and muscle mass achieved in young adulthood, and thus the rate of depletion in the reserve of these tissues during later ageing (46). Measures of muscle mass such as grip strength have been shown to be good predictors of later morbidity from a range of chronic conditions in addition to musculoskeletal problems (47).

MATERNAL GESTATIONAL VITAMIN D SUPPLEMENTATION AS A ROUTE TO OSTEOPOROSIS PREVENTION IN THE OFFSPRING

Maternal vitamin D supplementation during pregnancy serves as an illustrative example of an intervention early in life which may improve bone mass of the offspring. Thus the link between early development and adult osteoporosis risk was initially established in adult cohort studies such as that in Hertfordshire, and confirmed in a subsequent systematic review (48). More detailed skeletal phenotyping in such cohort studies demonstrated that a poor intrauterine environment (marked by low birthweight) was also associated with altered femoral geometry, compromised bone micro-architecture and reduced bone strength (49,50). Finally, analyses in the Helsinki cohort study suggested that an elevated risk of hip fracture in the offspring was associated with tall maternal stature, small body size at birth, and impaired childhood growth (51,52). More contemporaneous mother-offspring cohort studies in Southampton have demonstrated specific parental influences (maternal body build, smoking, physical activity and nutrition) on infant and childhood body composition, which were again confirmed in the Southampton Women's Survey (44,53). The overall quality of maternal nutrition before and during pregnancy as well as specific micronutrient deficiencies appeared to confer compromised skeletal development in the offspring (54). Among the latter, maternal vitamin D status appears to be a strong determinant of childhood bone and muscle mass independently of post-natal nutrition and physical activity (55,56). More detailed analyses of intrauterine bone growth using high-resolution ultrasound in the UK Southampton Women's Survey (SWS) revealed that maternal vitamin D insufficiency was linked to altered femoral morphology in utero (57), and that these influences might be mediated by DNA methylation in the promoter region of a gene (RXRA) whose product is heterodimeric with the vitamin D receptor and thereby intimately involved in vitamin D action (58). This combination of findings led to a systematic review of randomised controlled trials and cohort studies addressing vitamin D supplementation during pregnancy, which pointed at beneficial effects on maternal vitamin D status, umbilical venous calcium concentration and offspring bone mass and birthweight (56). The results of these original studies resulted in an alteration in public health policy to recommend a daily 400 IU vitamin D supplement to women during pregnancy (59,60). They also contributed to the justification of a large randomised controlled trial of maternal vitamin D supplementation during pregnancy (MAVIDOS) in which a 1000-IU daily supplement was contrasted with placebo, the primary outcome measure being bone mass of the offspring at birth. The recently published results from this trial suggested that supplementation was associated with a statistically significant and clinically relevant benefit to offspring bone mass for winter births (61); adjunctive analyses demonstrated that response to supplementation was influenced by genetic determinants of vitamin D metabolism and that supplementation altered the methylation profile in the promoter region of the RXRA gene. These observations are currently being tested in a second vitamin D trial (SPRING) (62) as well as through follow-up of the MAVIDOS offspring at 4 and 6 years of age.

CONCLUSION

As for other NCDs, there is good evidence that the risk of osteoporosis is partly set early in the lifecourse, and a range of factors relating to the developmental environment have been shown to be associated with early origins of the condition. Despite the well-established importance of the lifecourse concept to health (63), the challenge of how to utilise this concept in terms of early intervention remains. It may be that a combination of early life biomarkers, including epigenetic marks measured in accessible tissues, physiological functions such as grip strength, and assessment of bone density, will provide a valuable toolkit for assessment of later risk in time to institute a protective intervention. Such measures, collectively perhaps serving as an indication of intrinsic capacity, are likely in the foreseeable future only to be accessible in high resource settings. The problem of NCDs in low to middle income countries remains a major health, economic and humanitarian challenge.

ACKNOWLEDGEMENT

MAH is supported by the British Heart Foundation.

REFERENCES

1. Journal of Developmental Origins of Health and Disease. https://www.cambridge.org/core/journals/journal-of-developmental-origins-of-health-and-disease. Accessed 1 March 2017.
2. International Society of Developmental Origins of Health and Disease. https://dohadsoc.org/. Accessed 1 March 2017.
3. Hanson MA, Gluckman PD. Early developmental conditioning of later health and disease: Physiology or pathophysiology? *Physiolog Rev.* 2014;94:1027-76. doi:10.1152/physrev.00029.2013.
4. Dickinson H, Moss TJ, Gatford KL, Moritz KM, Akison L, Fullston T, et al. A review of fundamental principles for animal models of DOHaD research: An Australian perspective. *J Dev Orig Health Dis.* 2016 Oct;7(5):449-72.
5. Gage SH, Munafò MR, Davey Smith G. Causal inference in developmental origins of health and disease (DOHaD) research. *Ann Rev Psychol.* 2016 Jan 4;67:567-85.
6. Heindel JJ, Skalla LA, Joubert BR, Dilworth CH, Gray KA. Review of developmental origins of health and disease publications in environmental epidemiology. *Reprod Toxicol.* 2016 pii:s0890-6238(16)30413-0. doi:10.1016/j.reprodox.2016.11.011 Epub ahead of print.
7. Kuzawa CW, Gluckman PD, Hanson MA, Beedle AS. Evolution, developmental plasticity, and metabolic disease. In Stearns SC, Koella, editors. *Evolution in Health and Disease.* Oxford University Press; 2008:253-64.

8. Kuzawa CW, Quinn EA. Developmental origins of adult function and health: Evolutionary hypotheses. *Annu Rev Anthropol*. 2009 Oct 21;38:131-47.

9. Gilbert SF, Epel D. *Ecological Developmental Biology*. Sunderland MA: Sinauer; 2009:480.

10. Benyshek DC. The "early life" origins of obesity-related health disorders: New discoveries regarding the intergenerational transmission of developmentally programmed traits in the global cardiometabolic health crisis. *Am J Phys Anthropol*. 2013 Dec 1;152(S57):79-93.

11. Meloni M. How biology became social, and what it means for social theory. *Sociolog Rev*. 2014 Aug 1;62(3):593-614.

12. Barker DJ. *Mothers, Babies and Health in Later Life*. Elsevier Health Sciences; 1998.

13. Bertram CE, Hanson MA. Animal models and programming of the metabolic syndrome Type 2 diabetes. *Br Med Bull*. 2001 Nov 1;60(1):103-21.

14. Dickinson H, Moss TJ, Gatford KL, Moritz KM, Akison L, Fullston T, et al. A review of fundamental principles for animal models of DOHaD research: An Australian perspective. *J Dev Orig Health Dis*. 2016 Oct;7(5):449-72.

15. Inskip HM, Godfrey KM, Robinson SM, Law CM, Barker DJ, Cooper C, SWS Study Group. Cohort profile: The Southampton Women's Survey. *Int J Epidemiol*. 2006 Feb 1;35(1):42-8.

16. Jaddoe VW, van Duijn CM, Franco OH, van der Heijden AJ, van Ilzendoorn MH, de Jongste JC, et al. The Generation R Study: Design and cohort update 2012. *Eur J Epidemiol*. 2012 Sep 1;27(9):739-56.

17. Oken E, Baccarelli AA, Gold DR, Kleinman KP, Litonjua AA, De Meo D, et al. Cohort profile: Project Viva. *Int J Epidemiol*. 2014 Mar 16:dyu008.

18. Potdar RD, Sahariah SA, Gandhi M, Kehoe SH, Brown N, Sane H, et al. Improving women's diet quality preconceptionally and during gestation: Effects on birth weight and prevalence of low birth weight – A randomized controlled efficacy trial in India (Mumbai Maternal Nutrition Project). *Am J Clin Nutr*. 2014 Nov 1;100(5):1257-68.

19. World Health Organization. Global action plan for the prevention and control of noncommunicable diseases 2013–2020. WHO Press, Geneva, Switzerland, 2013.

20. World Health Organization. Noncommunicable diseases country profiles 2014. WHO Press, Geneva, Switzerland, 2014.

21. United Nations General Assembly. Political declaration of the high-level meeting of the general assembly on the prevention and control of noncommunicable diseases. New York: United Nations (2011). http://www.un.org/en/ga/ncdmeeting2011/pdf/NCD_draft_political_declaration.pdf. Accessed 9 November 2017.

22. United Nations. Sustainable Development Goals. http://www.un.org/sustainabledevelopment/sustainable-development-goals/. Accessed 7 March 2017.

23. Goran MI (ed). *Childhood Obesity: Causes, Consequences, and Intervention Approaches.* Boca Raton, FL: Taylor & Francis. 2017; ISBN: 9781498720656.

24. Green LR, Hester RL (eds). *Parental Obesity: Intergenerational Programming and Consequences.* Springer 2016. ISBN: 978-1-4939-6384-3.

25. Department of Health. Chief Medical Officer's Annual Report 2014: Health of the 51%: Women. www.gov.uk/government/uploads/system /uploads/attachment_data/file/484383/cmoreport-2014.pdf. Accessed 7 March 2017.

26. NCD Risk Factor Collaboration. Trends in adult body-mass index in 200 countries from 1975 to 2014: A pooled analysis of 1698 population-based measurement studies with 19·2 million participants. *Lancet.* 2016 Apr 8;387(10026):1377-96.

27. Hanson M, Barker M, Dodd JM, Kumanyika S, Norris S, Steegers E, et al. Interventions to prevent maternal obesity before conception, during pregnancy, and post partum. *Lancet Diabetes Endocrinol.* 2017 Jan 31;5(1):65-76.

28. Olsen MH, Angell SY, Asma S, Boutouyrie P, Burger D, Chirinos JA, et al. A call to action and a lifecourse strategy to address the global burden of raised blood pressure on current and future generations: The Lancet Commission on Hypertension. *Lancet.* 2016; 388: 2665-712.

29. Reynolds RM, Allan KM, Raja EA, Bhattacharya S, McNeill G, Hannaford PD, et al. Maternal obesity during pregnancy and premature mortality from cardiovascular event in adult offspring: Follow-up of 1 323 275 person years. *BMJ.* 2013 Aug 13;347:f4539.

30. World Health Organization. Global Strategy for Women's, Children's and Adolescent's Health 2016-2030. http://www.who.int/life-course/partners /global-strategy/en/. Accessed 7 March 2017.

31. Patton GC, Sawyer SM, Santelli JS, Ross DA, Afifi R, Allen NB, et al. Our future: A Lancet commission on adolescent health and wellbeing. *Lancet.* 2016 Jun 11;387(10036):2423-78.

32. United Nations. Convention on the Rights of the Child. http://www.unhcr .org/uk/4d9474b49.pdf. Accessed 7 March 2017.

33. Office of the High Commissioner for Human Rights. Adolescent Health and Development in the Context of the Convention of the Rights of the Child. http://www.ohchr.org/Documents/Issues/Women/WRGS/Health /GC4.pdf. Accessed 7 March 2017.

34. Twig G, Kark JD. Body-mass index in adolescence and cardiovascular death in adulthood. *N Engl J Med.* 2016 Sep 29;375(13):1300-1.

35. Gluckman PD, Hanson MA, Bateson P, Beedle AS, Law CM, Bhutta ZA, et al. Towards a new developmental synthesis: Adaptive developmental plasticity and human disease. *Lancet.* 2009 May 9;373(9675):1654.

36. García JL, Heckman JJ, Leaf DE, Prados MJ. The Life-cycle Benefits of an Influential Early Childhood Program. National Bureau of Economic Research; 2016 Dec 29.

37. Britto PR, Lye sj, Proulx K, Yousafzai AK, Matthews SG, Vaivada T, et al. Early Childhood Interventions Review Group, for the Lancet Early Childhood Development Series Steering Committee. Nurturing care: Promoting early childhood development. *Lancet*. 2017;389(10064), 91-102.

38. United Nations Systems Standing Committee on Nutrition. The UN Decade of Action on Nutrition 2016-2025. https://www.unscn.org/en/topics /un-decade-of-action-on-nutrition. Accessed 7 March 2017.

39. World Health Organization. Commission on Ending Childhood Obesity (ECHO). http://www.who.int/end-childhood-obesity/final-report/en/. Accessed 7 March 2017.

40. World Health Organization. Executive Board 140th Session. http://apps .who.int/gb/ebwha/pdf_files/EB140/B140_1-en.pdf. Accessed 7 March 2017.

41. Hanson MA, Bardsley A, De-Regil LM, Moore SE, Oken E, Poston L, et al. The International Federation of Gynecology and Obstetrics (FIGO) recommendations on adolescent, preconception, and maternal nutrition: "Think Nutrition First". *Int J Gynecol Obstet*. 2015 Oct 1;131(S4).

42. Dennison EM, Syddall HE, Sayer AA, Gilbody HJ, Cooper C. Birth weight and weight at 1 year are independent determinants of bone mass in the seventh decade: The Hertfordshire Cohort Study. *Pediatr Res*. 2005 Apr 1;57(4):582-6.

43. Dennison EM, Arden NK, Keen RW, Syddall H, Day IN, Spector TD, et al. Birthweight, vitamin D receptor genotype and the programming of osteoporosis. *Paediatr Perinat Epidemiol*. 2001 Jul 1;15(3):211-9.

44. Godfrey K, Walker-Bone K, Robinson S, Taylor P, Shore S, Wheeler T, et al. Neonatal bone mass: Influence of parental birthweight, maternal smoking, body composition, and activity during pregnancy. *J Bone Miner Res*. 2001 Sep 1;16(9):1694-703.

45. Cooper C, Cawley M, Bhalla A, Egger P, Ring F, Morton L, et al. Childhood growth, physical activity, and peak bone mass in women. *J Bone Miner Res*. 1995 Jun 1;10(6):940-7.

46. Hanson MA, Cooper C, Aihie Sayer A, Eendebak RJ, Clough GF, Beard JR. Developmental aspects of a life course approach to healthy ageing. *J Physiol*. 2016 Apr 15;594(8):2147-60.

47. Leong DP, Teo KK, Rangarajan S, Lopez-Jaramillo P, Avezum A, Orlandini A, et al. Prognostic value of grip strength: Findings from the Prospective Urban Rural Epidemiology (PURE) study. *Lancet*. 2015 Jul 24;386(9990):266-73.

48. Baird J, Kurshid MA, Kim M, Harvey N, Dennison E, Cooper C. Does birthweight predict bone mass in adulthood? A systematic review and meta-analysis. *Osteoporos Int*. 2011 May;22(5):1323-34.

49. Oliver H, Jameson KA, Sayer AA, Cooper C, Dennison EM. Growth in early life predicts bone strength in late adulthood: The Hertfordshire Cohort Study. *Bone*. 2007;41(3):400-5.

50. Harvey N, Dennison E, Cooper C. Osteoporosis: A lifecourse approach. *J Bone Miner Res*. 2014 Sep;29(9):1917-25.

51. Cooper C, Eriksson JG, Forsen T, Osmond C, Tuomilehto J, Barker DJ. Maternal height, childhood growth and risk of hip fracture in later life: A longitudinal study. *Osteoporos Int.* 2001;12(8):623-9.

52. Javaid MK, Eriksson JG, Kajantie E, Forsen T, Osmond C, Barker DJ, et al. Growth in childhood predicts hip fracture risk in later life. *Osteoporos Int.* 2011;22(1):69-73.

53. Harvey NC, Javaid MK, Arden NK, Poole JR, Crozier SR, Robinson SM, et al. Maternal predictors of neonatal bone size and geometry: The Southampton Women's Survey. *J Dev Orig Health Dis.* 2010;1(1):35-41.

54. Cole ZA, Gale CR, Javaid MK, Robinson SM, Law C, Boucher BJ, et al. Maternal dietary patterns during pregnancy and childhood bone mass: A longitudinal study. *J Bone Miner Res.* 2009;24(4):663-8.

55. Javaid MK, Crozier SR, Harvey NC, Gale CR, Dennison EM, Boucher BJ, et al. Maternal vitamin D status during pregnancy and childhood bone mass at age 9 years: A longitudinal study. *Lancet.* 2006;367(9504):36-43.

56. Harvey NC, Holroyd C, Ntani G, Javaid K, Cooper P, Moon R, et al. Vitamin D supplementation in pregnancy: A systematic review. *Health Technol Assess.* 2014 Jul;18(45):1-190.

57. Mahon P, Harvey N, Crozier S, Inskip H, Robinson S, Arden N, et al. Low maternal vitamin D status and fetal bone development: Cohort study. *J Bone Miner Res.* 2010;25(1):14-9.

58. Harvey NC, Sheppard A, Godfrey KM, McLean C, Garratt E, Ntani G, et al. Childhood bone mineral content is associated with methylation status of the RXRA promoter at birth. *J Bone Miner Res.* 2014 Mar;29(3):600-7.

59. UK DH. The Pregnancy Book 2009. http://webarchive.nationalarchives .gov.uk/+/www.dh.gov.uk/en/Publicationsandstatistics/Publications/Publi cationsPolicyandGuidance/DH_107302. Accessed 17 May 2017.

60. NICE. Antenatal care for uncomplicated pregnancies. Clinical guideline. (CG62). 2008. https://www.nice.org.uk/guidance/cg62/resources/antenatal -care-for-uncomplicated-pregnancies-pdf-975564597445. Accessed 17 May 2017.

61. Cooper C, Harvey NC, Bishop NJ, Kennedy S, Papageorghiou AT, Schoenmakers I, et al. Maternal gestational vitamin D supplementation and offspring bone health (MAVIDOS): A multicentre, double-blind, randomised placebo-controlled trial. *Lancet Diabetes Endocrinol.* 2016 May;4(5):393-402.

62. Baird J, Barker M, Harvey NC, Lawrence W, Vogel C, Jarman M, et al. Southampton Pregnancy Intervention for the Next Generation (SPRING): Protocol for a randomised controlled trial. *Trials.* 2016 Oct 12;17(1):493.

63. Kuh D, Cooper R, Hardy R, Richards M, Ben-Shlomo Y (eds). *A Life Course Approach to Healthy Ageing.* Oxford UK: Oxford University Press; 2013 Dec 19.

3

Early growth, bone development and risk of adult fracture

MICHAEL A CLYNES, NICHOLAS C HARVEY
AND ELAINE M DENNISON

INTRODUCTION

There are two principal factors that determine the risk of fracture: the mechanical strength of bone and the strength of the forces applied to it. The strength of a bone is directly related to 'bone mass', a term which describes a composite measure with contributions from bone size and volumetric bone mineral density (BMD). It has been well established that the bone mass of an individual in later life is determined by the peak bone mass attained during growth of the skeleton and, to a lesser extent, the rate of bone loss thereafter. Thus peak bone mass is a major determinant of risk of osteoporosis in old age, and there is increasing evidence that factors affecting bone mineral accrual in younger life may therefore influence peak bone mass, and fracture risk in older age (1). In a phenomenon known as 'tracking', the skeletal growth trajectory is determined early in life. Subsequently, a child's size relative to their peers remains fairly constant until they reach adulthood (see Chapter 9), shown graphically in Figure 3.1.

Osteoporosis is one of several diseases, including coronary heart disease, hypertension, type 2 diabetes and osteoarthritis, for which a low birthweight is

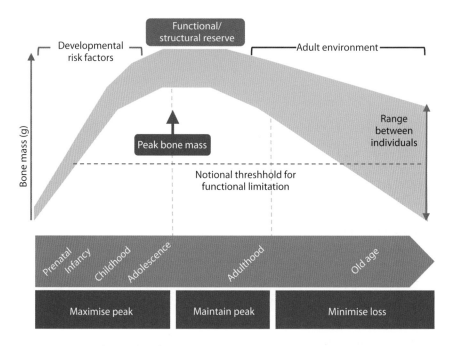

Figure 3.1 Development of bone mass over the lifecourse. Bone mass increases from the intrauterine period to a peak in early adulthood, with a decline thereafter. Modulation of the growth trajectory early in life may influence the magnitude of peak bone mass; intervention to reduce the rate of post-peak bone loss may be appropriate in older age. (Adapted with permission from Cooper C and Melton LJ, *Trends Endocrinol Metab.* 1992 Aug;3(6):224-9.)

predictive of the development of the disease in later life (2). Whilst genotype may explain a substantial proportion of the variation in adult bone mass, evidence is accruing that interaction between the genome and the environment during the intrauterine period and early childhood is critical for setting the growth trajectory and therefore bone mass and later skeletal health (2). This process has been termed 'programming'. Much of the original work on programming was conducted by Barker and colleagues (see Chapters 2 and 14), who reported an association between coronary heart disease and low birth weight (used as a proxy for fetal growth); the term *developmental origins of health and disease* (DOHaD) was subsequently established.

It is clear that skeletal health in later life can be profoundly influenced by early growth. This chapter discusses the contribution of early growth to the developmental origins of osteoporosis, detailing large epidemiological studies and exploring potential underlying mechanisms.

GROWTH AND SKELETAL DEVELOPMENT (1)

Historical perspective

One of the earliest descriptions of growth through childhood was made by Count Philibert Gueneau de Montbeillard, charting his son's increase in height over 18 years from 1759 to 1777, and recorded by Georges-Louis Leclerc, Comte de Buffon, in the French *Histoire Naturelle*. A plot of absolute height, and height gain per year, demonstrated rapid change over the first 2 years of life but with progressive deceleration over this period, a relatively stable rate of growth until puberty, followed by a rapid acceleration and then deceleration over the later pubertal period. The growth patterns so documented by Montbeillard have been confirmed by subsequent investigators, in particular John Tanner, who undertook much of the seminal work in this area (3–5). Assessing growth in postnatal life is relatively straightforward, notwithstanding logistic issues of cohort generation and repeatability of measurements; attempting to produce the same sort of graphical representation of growth in utero is much more problematic. Until the advent of ultrasound scanning, this work inevitably had to rely on cross-sectional data. Indeed, an early paper from Tanner, in which growth is described across the intrauterine and into the postnatal period, relied on separate pre- and postnatal datasets. The prenatal data were cross-sectional, based on measurements of neonates born at different gestations, and the postnatal measurements were longitudinal. Cross-sectional measurements of size at different gestations, rather than longitudinal measurements within subjects, can lead to erroneous conclusions regarding growth trajectory, tending to overly smooth individual curves. More recently longitudinal data have been published, and these will be described in subsequent sections.

The pattern of growth described by Tanner suggests that linear growth velocity increases throughout the first half of pregnancy and then slows; velocity of weight gain appears to slow from around 32 weeks (3–5). This growth velocity deceleration as delivery is approached is an important physiological happening, as unchecked growth might lead to a baby unable to exit through the birth canal. This phenomenon is known as 'maternal constraint' and is poorly understood in mechanistic terms (see Chapters 2 and 14). It is, however, clearly a powerful process: a cross between a Shetland pony and a shire horse results in the birth of a small foal when the Shetland pony is the mother, and a large foal when the shire horse is the mother (6); interestingly the respective offspring are the same size when fully grown, which is midway between the two parents. This graphic illustration from an animal model is consistent with human data, suggesting that there is a substantial environmental contribution to birthweight.

Prospective assessments of early growth and postnatal bone size, mineralisation and geometry

The use of high-resolution ultrasound measurements during pregnancy have enabled much more detailed, and, importantly, longitudinal assessment of fetal growth to be made, and to be related to later outcomes such as bone mineral and body composition (7–9). The UK Southampton Women's Survey (SWS) (10) is particularly well set up to investigate relationships between early growth and childhood bone mass. It is a unique prospective population-based cohort study of 12,583 initially non-pregnant women aged 20 to 34 years, and representative of the UK population. Women were assessed in detail at study entry in terms of diet, lifestyle, body build, physical activity, health and medications, and venous blood was collected. Similar assessments were conducted in early (11 weeks) and late (34 weeks) gestation in those (n = 3159) who became pregnant. High-resolution ultrasound scans were obtained at 11, 19 and 34 weeks' gestation with measurements of indices such as crown–rump length, head, chest, abdominal circumferences and femur length performed according to published guidelines by two trained operators. Offspring have been measured in detail at birth and then at 6 months and 1, 2 and 3 years. Consecutive samples of around 1000 children have undergone dual-energy X-ray absorptiometry (DXA) (whole body and lumbar spine, and from 4 years onwards, also both hips) and anthropometric assessments at birth, 4 and 6 years, with visits at 8 and 11 years ongoing. Peripheral quantitative computed tomography (pQCT) measurements of tibial bone strength are available at 6 years.

The choice of statistical methods with which to model growth continues to be widely debated, and different methods (e.g. conditional regression, fitted linear or polynomial equations, latent growth curve modelling) all have their merits. The time points at which data are recorded may impose some restriction on the method chosen; for example fitted polynomial equations are more appropriate for data recorded at many, and potentially overlapping, points across time. In the SWS analyses, where assessments are undertaken at discrete time points, conditional growth modelling based on variables converted to within group z-scores was employed. The technique makes no assumptions about segmentation or shape of the growth trajectory, and uses regression-derived residuals to generate mutually independent variables describing growth velocity across successive periods; for example 11 to 19 weeks, 19 to 34 weeks, birth to 1 year.

Data from the SWS have informed three areas of investigation: (i) differential effects of growth on bone size and BMD; (ii) specific timing of relationships; and (iii) effects on hip geometry. In a subset of 380 mother-child pairs with complete data for femur length and abdominal circumference at 19 and 34 weeks, together with DXA indices at 4 years, differential relationships were observed between growth measurements and childhood bone mass depending on adjustment for body size (7). Thus the velocity of late pregnancy fetal abdominal growth was positively associated with childhood bone mineral content (BMC) after adjustment for body size (BMC adjusted for bone area [BA] height and weight: r = 0.15, p = 0.004) but not with skeletal size (BA: r = 0.06, p = 0.21). In contrast, the velocity of late pregnancy fetal femur growth was positively associated with 4-year skeletal size (BA: r = 0.30, p < 0.0001) but not with size-corrected BMC (r = 0.03, p = 0.51). Given that femur length is a component of skeletal size, it is not surprising that it is strongly associated with whole body bone area at 4 years, and less so with BMC adjusted for body size (which also gives an indirect indication of volumetric mineralisation). However, the associations between abdominal circumference growth and size-corrected BMC are intriguing, and suggest that changes in the subcomponents of the ultrasound measure – for example liver size or subcutaneous fat stores – might influence accrual of volumetric BMD. The involvement of adipose tissue is supported by findings from an earlier study in which umbilical cord venous serum concentrations of leptin were positively associated with DXA-assessed size-corrected BMC in the neonate (11) and the known effects of leptin on bone formation; in contrast, umbilical cord venous serum concentrations of IGF1, a potent osteoblast stimulus produced in the fetal liver, have been associated with neonatal bone size, but not density, in a similar study design (12).

This work was extended to explore the temporal relationships between different phases of intrauterine and postnatal growth, and postnatal bone mass at birth and 4 years, using abdominal circumference, which can be measured at all three timepoints (11, 19 and 34 weeks' gestation, unlike femur length which can be assessed from 19 weeks onwards), as the primary growth measure (9). This measure was also available postnatally at birth and 1, 2 and 3 years. Linear growth was assessed by femur length at 19 and 34 weeks and then postnatally by length (birth and 1 year) and height (2, 3 and 4 years old).

Relationships differed according to timing in pregnancy, with abdominal circumference growth in late pregnancy strongly related to bone mass at birth, but less so with bone mass at 4 years. In contrast, abdominal circumference growth in early pregnancy was more strongly related to bone mass at 4 years than at birth. For linear growth, the strongest associations with bone mass at 4 years were for growth in late pregnancy and in the first 2 years of postnatal life. Indeed the proportion of children changing their position in the length distribution at each postnatal time point progressively decreased, consistent with the gradual settling onto a more sustained growth trajectory. This pattern of perturbation of growth in late pregnancy and early infancy, with gradual settling onto a longer-term trajectory, was confirmed in a study relating early linear growth to proximal femoral geometry at 6 years in Southampton Women's Survey children (8). Here, in 493 children assessed by DXA at 6 years, hip strength analysis was related to conditional measures of linear growth from 11 weeks' gestation to 6 years postnatal life, with the strongest relationships for growth in late pregnancy and infancy. Figure 3.2 shows the standardized regression coefficients for linear growth at each time interval as predictors of narrow femoral neck section modulus (a measure of bending strength).

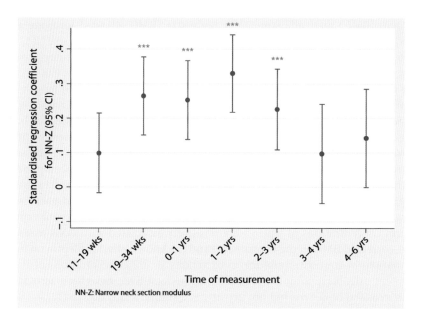

NN-Z: Narrow neck section modulus

Figure 3.2 Linear growth from late pregnancy into childhood and narrow femoral neck section modulus at six years. Data are standardised regression coefficients showing the SD change in outcome per SD change in growth over each time period. The measures of linear size are crown–rump length (11 weeks' gestation), femur length (19 and 34 weeks' gestation), crown–heel length (birth and 1 year postnatally) and standing height British Growth Foundation z-scores (2 to 6 years postnatally). (Reproduced with permission from Harvey NC et al. *Pediatr Res.* 2013 Jul 15.)

Critical growth periods for later bone development

These observations support the earlier findings documented by Tanner (3–5), and the models of Karlberg (13), but here for the first time, such associations have been documented using objective measures in a truly prospective cohort. These results would be consistent with the notion that there may be critical periods where growth velocity relates very strongly to longer term measures of bone development, and thus offer potential opportunities for early intervention to optimize skeletal strength. These findings have been supported by studies from birth cohorts elsewhere. In Generation R, a mother-offspring cohort in Rotterdam, the Netherlands, fetal weight gain and catch-up in weight were associated with BMD at the whole body site at 6 months (14). Furthermore, children remaining in the lowest tertile of weight from birth to 6 months had a much higher risk of having low BMD at the whole body site at 6 months of age. In a Norwegian cohort, fetal femur length was measured using 2D ultrasound in 625 pregnancies. Consistent with the pattern of altered growth velocity in late pregnancy, femur length z-scores measured between 10 and 19 weeks were progressively less strongly correlated with later measurements (r = 0.59 [weeks 20–26], r = 0.45 [weeks 27–33] and r = 0.32 [weeks 34–39]; all p < 0.001) (15).

Early growth and adult bone mass

These studies of growth in early life and childhood bone indices shed light on previous studies which related indirect measures of growth such as birthweight and weight at 1 year to measures of adult bone mass, in large cohorts of individuals where birth/childhood records have been preserved. The first such study to demonstrate a link between the development of osteoporosis and weight in infancy studied 153 women born in Bath (UK) during 1968–1969 who were traced and studied at 21 years of age (16). Cooper and colleagues obtained data on childhood growth from linked birth and school records and found statistically significant (p < 0.05) associations between BMC at the lumbar spine and femoral neck, and weight at 1 year. Furthermore, these relationships were independent of adult weight and body mass index. The observation that weight in infancy influences adult bone mass was replicated in a second cohort of individuals from Hertfordshire (UK). In this study it was obseved that there was a significant association between weight at 1 year and adult bone area at the spine and hip (p < 0.005). There was also a signifcant relationship between weight at year one and BMC at both these sites (p < 0.02). These observations remained significant following adjustment for potential confounding lifestyle factors which could affect bone mass in adulthood (physical activity, dietary calcium intake, smoking, alcohol consumption) (17). Associations between birthweight or weight at 1 year and later BMC have been confirmed across a range of studies internationally and summarised in a recent systematic review and meta-analysis (18). A later study utilised pQCT to evaluate cortical and trabecular bone density, strength-strain index and fracture load in the distal radius and tibia (19). A strong association was found between birthweight, weight at 1 year, and bone width, length and area at the tibia (and to a lesser extent proximal radius) in both sexes. An association was also observed between birthweight and weight at 1 year, with fracture load and strength–strain index at the tibia and proximal radius. Again, these observations remained significant after adjustment for confounders (age, body mass index, social class, cigarette smoking, alcohol consumption, physical activity, dietary calcium intake and hormone replacement therapy use among women).

Early growth and risk of adult hip fracture

Data from adult cohorts in which birth records exist clearly demonstrate the implications of such findings for fracture risk: in a large Finnish cohort, poor growth in both early and later postnatal life was associated with increased risk of adult hip fracture 7 decades later (20,21) (Figure 3.3). This finding is complemented by results from the Hertfordshire cohort demonstrating positive associations between early weight and femoral cross-sectional area, independent of femoral neck length. Taken together such results support a link between early growth, femoral geometry and risk of adult hip fracture (22), and critically, potential windows of opportunity for intervention early in life to optimise skeletal development.

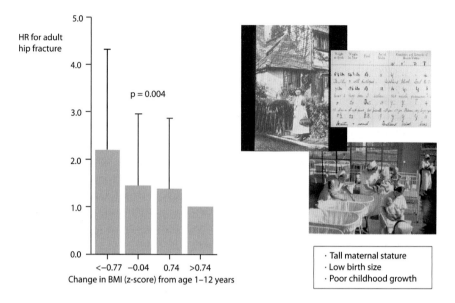

Figure 3.3 Poor growth in utero and childhood predict later risk of hip fracture (Helsinki and Hertfordshire cohort studies). Figure demonstrates data from the original Hertfordshire birth ledgers together with hazard ratio (HR) for adult hip fracture by quartile of change in BMI z-score from age 1 to 12 years in the Helsinki cohort. (Data from Javaid MK et al. *Osteoporos Int.* 2011;22(1):69-73; reproduced with permission from Harvey NC et al. *J Bone Miner Res.* 2014 Sep;29(9):1917-25.)

CONCLUSION

Our understanding of the pathogenesis of osteoporosis has advanced greatly over the past 2 decades. There is now compelling evidence to suggest that osteoporosis has developmental origins and that there are significant environmental factors, in addition to genetic inheritance, which determine our risk of developing the disease. This underlines the importance of adopting preventative strategies for osteoporosis at all stages of the lifecourse including the in-utero environment. It is evident that optimising both maternal and infant nutrition are essential strategies for decreasing future osteoporosis risk. The mechanisms through which our skeletal health is programmed, which we are now beginning to elucidate, could be key to the development of future preventative strategies.

ACKNOWLEDGEMENT

Parts of this chapter are adapted with permission from Harvey et al. (1).

REFERENCES

1. Harvey N, Dennison E, Cooper C. Osteoporosis: A lifecourse approach. *J Bone Miner Res.* 2014 Sep;29(9):1917-25. PubMed PMID: 24861883. Epub 2014/05/28. eng.

2. Gluckman PD, Hanson MA, Cooper C, Thornburg KL. Effect of in utero and early-life conditions on adult health and disease. *N Engl J Med.* 2008;359(1):61-73.

3. Tanner JM. *Growth before birth.* In: *Foetus into Man: Physical Growth from Conception to Maturity.* 2nd ed. Ware: Castlemead Publications; 1989:36-50.

4. Tanner JM. The interaction of heredity and environment in the control of growth. In: *Foetus into Man: Physical Growth from Conception to Maturity.* 2nd ed. Ware: Castlemead Publications; 1989:119-64.

5. Tanner JM. The organisation of the growth process. In: *Foetus into Man: Physical Growth from Conception to Maturity.* 2nd ed. Ware: Castlemead Publications; 1989:165-77.

6. Walton A, Hammond J. The maternal effects on growth and conformation in Shire horse-Shetland pony crosses. *Proc R Soc Lond (Biol).* 1938;125: 311-35.

7. Harvey N, Mahon P, Robinson S, Nisbet C, Javaid M, Crozier S, et al. Different indices of fetal growth predict bone size and volumetric density at 4 years old. *J Bone Miner Res.* 2010;25:920-27.

8. Harvey NC, Cole ZA, Crozier SR, Ntani G, Mahon PA, Robinson SM, et al. Fetal and infant growth predict hip geometry at six years old: Findings from the Southampton Women's Survey. *Pediatr Res.* 2013 Jul 15. PubMed PMID: 23857297. Epub 2013/07/17. eng.

9. Harvey NC, Mahon PA, Kim M, Cole ZA, Robinson SM, Javaid K, et al. Intrauterine growth and postnatal skeletal development: Findings from the Southampton Women's Survey. *Paediatr Perinat Epidemiol.* 2012 Jan;26(1):34-44. PubMed PMID: 22150706. Epub 2011/12/14. eng.

10. Inskip HM, Godfrey KM, Robinson SM, Law CM, Barker DJ, Cooper C. Cohort profile: The Southampton Women's Survey. *Int J Epidemiol.* 2005. 2006 Feb;35(1):42-8.

11. Javaid MK, Godfrey KM, Taylor P, Robinson SM, Crozier SR, Dennison EM, et al. Umbilical cord leptin predicts neonatal bone mass. *Calcif Tissue Int.* 2005 May;76(5):341-7. PubMed PMID: 15864467. Epub 2005/05/03. eng.

12. Javaid MK, Godfrey KM, Taylor P, Shore SR, Breier B, Arden NK, et al. Umbilical venous IGF-1 concentration, neonatal bone mass, and body composition. *J Bone Miner Res.* 2004;19(1):56-63.

13. Karlberg J, Engstrom I, Karlberg P, Fryer JG. Analysis of linear growth using a mathematical model. I. From birth to three years. *Acta Paediatr Scand.* 1987;76(3):478-88.

14. Ay L, Jaddoe VW, Hofman A, Moll HA, Raat H, Steegers EA, et al. Foetal and postnatal growth and bone mass at 6 months: The Generation R Study. *Clin Endocrinol (Oxf)*. 2011 Feb;74(2):181-90. PubMed PMID: 21050252. Epub 2010/11/06. eng.

15. Bjornerem A, Johnsen SL, Nguyen TV, Kiserud T, Seeman E. The shifting trajectory of growth in femur length during gestation. *J Bone Miner Res*. 2010 May;25(5):1029-33. PubMed PMID: 19929433. Epub 2009/11/26. eng.

16. Cooper C, Cawley M, Bhalla A, Egger P, Ring F, Morton L, et al. Childhood growth, physical activity, and peak bone mass in women. *J Bone Miner Res*. 1995;10(6):940-7.

17. Dennison EM, Aihie-Sayer A, Syddall H, Arden N, Gilbody H, Cooper C. Birthweight is associated with bone mass in the seventh decade: The Hertfordshire 31-39 Study. *Pediatr Res*. 2003;53 S25A.

18. Baird J, Kurshid MA, Kim M, Harvey N, Dennison E, Cooper C. Does birthweight predict bone mass in adulthood? A systematic review and meta-analysis. *Osteoporos Int*. 2011 May;22(5):1323-34. PubMed PMID: 20683711. Epub 2010/08/05. eng.

19. Oliver H, Jameson KA, Sayer AA, Cooper C, Dennison EM. Growth in early life predicts bone strength in late adulthood: The Hertfordshire cohort study. *Bone*. 2007;41(3):400-5.

20. Cooper C, Eriksson JG, Forsen T, Osmond C, Tuomilehto J, Barker DJ. Maternal height, childhood growth and risk of hip fracture in later life: A longitudinal study. *Osteoporos Int J*. 9100105. 2001;12(8):623-9.

21. Javaid MK, Eriksson JG, Kajantie E, Forsen T, Osmond C, Barker DJ, et al. Growth in childhood predicts hip fracture risk in later life. *Osteoporos Int*. 2011 Jan;22(1):69-73. PubMed PMID: 20379699.

22. Javaid MK, Lekamwasam S, Clark J, Dennison EM, Syddall HE, Loveridge N, et al. Infant growth influences proximal femoral geometry in adult-hood. *J Bone Miner Res*. 2006;21(4):508-12.

4

Maternal nutrition, lifestyle and anthropometry during pregnancy and offspring bone development

REBECCA J MOON AND NICHOLAS C HARVEY

INTRODUCTION

An ageing population will lead to an ever-increasing burden of osteoporosis. Indeed worldwide, hip fracture incidence has been predicted to rise from 1.7 million in 1990 to 6.3 million in 2050 (1). As such, new strategies aimed at primary prevention of osteoporosis are needed. In adults, fracture risk is strongly associated with bone mineral density (BMD) (2), and thus approaches aimed at increasing BMD early in life might be beneficial. There is increasing recognition that the in utero environment can modify fetal bone development with persisting effects into later childhood (the concept of Developmental Origins of Health and Disease is described in more detail in Chapters 2 and 14). This chapter discusses the relationships between maternal dietary and lifestyle characteristics and offspring bone mineralisation.

FETAL BONE DEVELOPMENT

At birth, the average weight of an infant is 3.0 to 3.5 kg, of which approximately 66 g is bone mineral, therefore representing around 2% of body weight (3). Bone development begins from 8 to 12 weeks' gestation by endochondral ossification to form the long bones and intramembranous ossification to form the flat bones such as the skull. Although a cartilaginous bone model is laid down early in development of the long bones, the principal period of bone mineral deposition is during the third trimester. Skeletal mineralisation in the fetus is primarily determined by fetal plasma calcium ion (Ca^{2+}) concentration, which is dependent on the active transfer of Ca^{2+} from the maternal to the fetal circulation by the placenta and fetal calcitropic hormones, including parathyroid hormone (PTH) and parathyroid hormone–related peptide (PTHrP) (4,5). Fetal plasma Ca^{2+} is maintained at a higher concentration than that in the mother (6), which is in part dependent on increased maternal calcium absorption from the gut. Thus it could be postulated that limited availability of the substrates for bone development due to nutritional depletion or impaired placental transfer is likely to impact negatively on fetal bone development. Indeed placental volume at 19 weeks' gestation has been positively associated with offspring whole body bone area (BA), bone mineral content (BMC) and areal BMD (7).

MATERNAL DIET AND OFFSPRING BONE MINERALISATION

Dietary quality

The Princess Anne Hospital Study was one of the earliest mother-offspring birth cohort studies to examine the associations between maternal diet and lifestyle and offspring bone development. In this study, 198 women from Southampton, UK had diet assessed by a food frequency questionnaire (FFQ) at 15 and 32 weeks' gestation. A dietary score was calculated to quantify the consistency of the dietary intake with recommendations for a healthy diet. A more prudent diet in late pregnancy, characterised by greater intakes of fruit, vegetables, wholemeal bread, rice and pasta, yoghurt and breakfast cereals and low intakes of chips, roast potatoes, processed meat, sugar, crisps and soft drinks, was positively associated with offspring whole body and lumbar spine (LS) BMC and areal BMD (aBMD) measured by dual-energy X-ray absorptiometry (DXA) at 9 years of age. This association remained statistically significant after adjustment for maternal social class, educational achievement, anthropometry and smoking status. Whole body BMC and BA were 11% and 8% higher, respectively, in the children born to mothers in the highest quartile of prudent diet score compared to those in the lowest quartile (8). These findings are supported by recently published data from the Danish National Birth Cohort, which included over 50,000 mother-offspring pairs. Using a FFQ undertaken in mid-pregnancy, a Western diet defined as a high intake of meat, potatoes and white bread, and low intake of vegetables, fruit and cereals, was associated with a higher risk of forearm fracture during childhood in the offspring (9).

Individual dietary components

A number of studies have attempted to elucidate whether individual dietary components are associated with offspring bone development. Unsurprisingly, given the importance to bone mineral accrual, the most frequently studied of these are calcium and vitamin D. The relationships between in utero vitamin D exposure and prenatal bone development are discussed in Chapter 4.

There have been four mother-offspring birth-cohort studies assessing the associations between maternal calcium intake and offspring bone development (10–14). The findings of these are inconsistent, but this could reflect the variations in the populations studied, including both developed and developing countries, the timing of calcium intake assessment and the age at which the offspring were studied. In the Pune Maternal Nutritional Study (India), maternal calcium intake was assessed at 18 and 28 weeks' gestation by FFQ, with DXA assessment of 698 children at 6 years of age. In this population, in which calcium intake is typically low, intake at both 18 and 28 weeks' gestation was associated with offspring whole body BMC and BMD, but these relationships were attenuated in multivariate analysis. However, milk intake at 28 weeks' gestation accounted for 1.1% of the variance in whole body BMD in multivariate analysis (10). Two large European birth cohort studies including approximately 3000 mother-offspring pairs have also studied this relationship. The Generation R project in The Netherlands assessed maternal calcium intake in the first trimester with offspring DXA at 6 years of age (11), and the Avon Longitudinal Study of Parents and Children (ALPSAC) determined maternal calcium intake at 32 weeks' gestation and assessed the offspring at 9 years of age (12). Despite these methodological differences, both studies did identify positive associations between maternal calcium intake and offspring whole body less head BMC and aBMD, but these did not remain significant in multivariate analysis. However, high collinearity between maternal calcium intake and other dietary factors was observed, which may have complicated the estimation of the contribution of each individual dietary component.

The few randomised control trials (RCT) of calcium supplementation in pregnancy have also reported inconsistent findings (15–17). The first of these was carried out in India in 1978 and included 78 women of low socioeconomic status. The women were randomised to 300 mg calcium per day, 600 mg calcium per day or placebo from 20 weeks' gestation. Neonatal BMD was determined by radiographic density from radiographs of the ulna, radius, tibia and fibula. Significant increases in this measurement were observed in the neonates born to mothers in both the calcium supplementation groups compared to the placebo group, but no difference between the two supplementation doses was observed (17). In contrast, two studies using DXA assessment of BMD in the offspring of mothers randomised to calcium supplementation did not find positive effects of supplementation. A randomised placebo controlled trial of 1500 mg/day calcium supplementation from 20 weeks' gestation in the Gambia, where calcium intake is typically very low, did not identify differences in infant whole body BMC or BMD at 2, 13 or 52 weeks post-delivery (18). Furthermore, calcium supplementation appeared to have a detrimental effect on maternal BMC, which was lower in the supplemented women than those randomised to placebo, when assessed at least 3 months after completion of breastfeeding (15). Similarly, supplementation of women in the United States to 2 g/day calcium from 22 weeks' gestation did not increase neonatal whole body or LS BMD in the offspring compared to placebo, except when only women in the lowest quintile of dietary calcium intake were considered (16). This therefore suggests that supplementation could be beneficial to offspring of mothers with the lowest levels of calcium intake, but as maternal DXA was not undertaken in this study, confirmation that detrimental effects on the maternal skeleton, such as those in the Gambian study, do not occur, is needed. However, this study would suggest that increasing calcium intake in women with an already sufficient dietary load may not be of benefit to fetal bone mineral accrual. As fetal plasma Ca^{2+} is tightly regulated by PTHrP and PTH, and placental transfer is an active process, transfer from the maternal to fetal circulation could already be saturated in those with sufficient dietary intake.

Several studies have also examined the relationships between other individual dietary components, including macronutrients and micronutrients (e.g. phosphorus, folate, magnesium) in pregnancy and offspring bone mass. Using the ALSPAC cohort, in univariate analysis, maternal fibre, protein, milk sugar, magnesium, phosphorous, potassium, zinc, iron, niacin and vitamin C intakes assessed by FFQ at 32 weeks' gestation were associated with offspring whole body minus head aBMD at 9 years of age. However, in multivariate analysis, only magnesium intake remained significantly positively associated. Although the effect size was small, with only approximately 1% difference in whole body aBMD between offspring of mothers in the highest and lowest tertile of intake (12), another analysis using the same ALSPAC cohort found a 0.6% difference in whole body aBMD between children that did and did not sustain a fracture in the subsequent 24 months after assessment at 9 years (19). This therefore suggests that even the small effect on aBMD observed in relation to maternal dietary factors might alter clinical outcomes for the offspring.

FFQs are limited in their accuracy by participant reporting and consistency of portion size. Therefore studies using serum measurements of micronutrients may be more reliable. The Southampton Women's Survey (SWS), a prospective mother-offspring pre-birth cohort study in Southampton, UK, has assessed the relationships between a number of maternal serum nutritional markers and offspring bone variables assessed by DXA. For example, positive associations were identified between maternal serum measurements of n-3 polyunsaturated fatty acids (PUFA), typically found in fish oils, at 34 weeks' gestation and offspring whole body minus head and LS BMC and BMD at 4 years of age in 727 mother-child pairs, replicating similar findings in animal studies (20). Maternal serum retinol at 34 weeks gestation was negatively associated with neonatal whole body BA and BMC, but not BMD, whereas serum beta-carotene was positively associated with these measures (21). Interestingly, this is consistent with the observed associations with hip fracture in older adults, with retinol intake being positively associated with fracture risk, but beta-carotene intake negatively associated (22). Nonetheless, replication of these findings in further cohorts is required before trials of supplementation can be considered.

SMOKING

Smoking during pregnancy has been linked to poorer placental function (23) and lower birth weight, and smoking in later life has been associated with increased fracture risk (24). However, the evidence linking gestational smoking to detrimental effects on offspring bone health is inconclusive. In the Princess Anne Hospital Study and SWS, reductions in neonatal whole body BMC and bone area of infants born to mothers who smoked during pregnancy compared to non-smoking mothers were observed (Figure 4.1) (25,26). However, bone mineral apparent density (BMAD), was not significantly different in one study (25), and the differences were no longer present after adjustment for infant length in the other (26), suggesting the effect of smoking on bone development is on overall skeletal size rather than mineralisation.

In contrast, a number of studies have suggested that children born to mothers who smoked in pregnancy have higher measures of BMC, BMD and BA during later childhood and adolescence, but that this association is mediated by the higher body weight observed in children born to mothers who smoked (27–30). There are limited data in relation to childhood fracture incidences, but in one study this did not differ according to maternal smoking status in pregnancy (30). However, obesity is more common in children born to mothers who smoked in pregnancy, and this may be detrimental to bone health in later life (31).

MATERNAL BODY COMPOSITION AND PHYSICAL ACTIVITY

In the SWS, both maternal height and triceps skinfold thickness, used as a measure of adiposity, were positively associated with offspring BMC and BA in the neonatal period (Figure 4.1). Whilst the association with triceps skinfold thickness was robust for adjustment for infant length, the association with maternal height was not, suggesting an association with mineralisation and not just skeletal size (26). In contrast, maternal walking speed in pregnancy, as a marker of physical activity, was negatively associated with BMC and BA, even after adjustment for infant length.

MATERNAL AGE

Advancing maternal age has been associated with lower lumbar spine BMD in young adult males in a birth cohort study in Sweden, after adjustment for a number of potential confounding factors including calcium intake, level of physical activity, height and weight, total body adipose tissue and lean mass and smoking status of the adult male, and parental socioeconomic status, maternal parity, paternal age, smoking in pregnancy, gestation at birth and birth length (32).

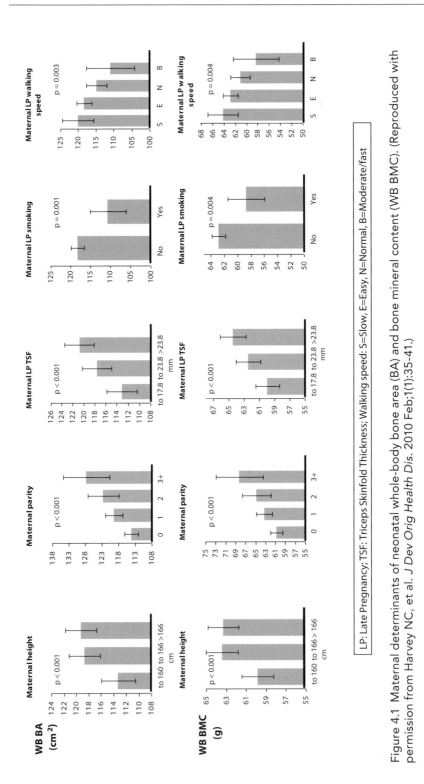

LP: Late Pregnancy; TSF: Triceps Skinfold Thickness; Walking speed: S=Slow, E=Easy, N=Normal, B=Moderate/fast

Figure 4.1 Maternal determinants of neonatal whole-body bone area (BA) and bone mineral content (WB BMC). (Reproduced with permission from Harvey NC, et al. *J Dev Orig Health Dis*. 2010 Feb;1(1):35-41.)

Using peripheral quantitative computed tomography (pQCT), maternal age was also negatively associated with endosteal and periosteal circumference of the non-dominant radius, but not with volumetric BMD (32). Nonetheless, bone size is also important to fracture risk.

CONCLUSIONS

Novel approaches to the primary prevention of osteoporosis are much needed, and thus the role of in utero factors in bone mass accrual should be considered. Many of the data relating maternal factors to offspring bone development are currently observational in nature and findings are inconsistent, but variations in methodological design – in particular timing of maternal and offspring assessment – limit comparison of studies. However, the observational data do highlight a need to explore this further, and randomised controlled trials of dietary supplementation are now required to be certain that the relationships are not due to unknown confounding and that the findings are not population-specific.

REFERENCES

1. Cooper C, Campion G, Melton LJ, 3rd. Hip fractures in the elderly: A world-wide projection. *Osteoporos Int.* 1992 Nov;2(6):285-9. PubMed PMID: 1421796. Epub 1992/11/01. eng.
2. Cummings SR, Black DM, Nevitt MC, Browner W, Cauley J, Ensrud K, et al. Bone density at various sites for prediction of hip fractures. The Study of Osteoporotic Fractures Research Group. *Lancet* (London, England). 1993 Jan 9;341(8837):72-5. PubMed PMID: 8093403. Epub 1993/01/09. eng.
3. Koo WW, Walters J, Bush AJ, Chesney RW, Carlson SE. Dual-energy X-ray absorptiometry studies of bone mineral status in newborn infants. *J Bone Miner Res.* 1996;11(7):997-1102.
4. Belkacemi L, Bedard I, Simoneau L, Lafond J. Calcium channels, transporters and exchangers in placenta: A review. *Cell Calcium.* 2005;37(1):1-8.
5. Kovacs CS, Chafe LL, Fudge NJ, Friel JK, Manley NR. PTH regulates fetal blood calcium and skeletal mineralization independently of PTHrP. *Endocrinology.* 2001;142(11):4983-93.
6. Forestier F, Daffos F, Rainaut M, Bruneau M, Trivin F. Blood chemistry of normal human fetuses at midtrimester of pregnancy. *Pediatr Res.* 1987;21(6):579-83.
7. Holroyd CR, Harvey NC, Crozier SR, Winder NR, Mahon PA, Ntani G, et al. Placental size at 19 weeks predicts offspring bone mass at birth: Findings from the Southampton Women's Survey. *Placenta.* 2012 Aug;33(8):623-9. PubMed PMID: 22640438. PubMed Central PMCID: Pmc3800076. Epub 2012/05/30. eng.
8. Cole ZA, Gale CR, Javaid MK, Robinson SM, Law C, Boucher BJ, et al. Maternal dietary patterns during pregnancy and childhood bone mass: A longitudinal study. *J Bone Miner Res.* 2009 Apr;24(4):663-8. PubMed PMID: 19049331. Epub 2008/12/04. eng.

9. Petersen SB, Rasmussen MA, Olsen SF, Vestergaard P, Molgaard C, Halldorsson TI, et al. Maternal dietary patterns during pregnancy in relation to offspring forearm fractures: Prospective study from the Danish National Birth Cohort. *Nutrients*. 2015 Apr;7(4):2382-400. PubMed PMID: 25849947. PubMed Central PMCID: Pmc4425150. Epub 2015/04/08. eng.

10. Ganpule A, Yajnik CS, Fall CH, Rao S, Fisher DJ, Kanade A, et al. Bone mass in Indian children – Relationships to maternal nutritional status and diet during pregnancy: The Pune Maternal Nutrition Study. *J Clin Endocrinol Metab*. 2006;91(8):2994-3001.

11. Heppe DH, Medina-Gomez C, Hofman A, Franco OH, Rivadeneira F, Jaddoe VW. Maternal first-trimester diet and childhood bone mass: The Generation R Study. *Am J Clin Nutr*. 2013 Jul;98(1):224-32. PubMed PMID: 23719545. Epub 2013/05/31. eng.

12. Tobias JH, Steer CD, Emmett PM, Tonkin RJ, Cooper C, Ness AR. Bone mass in childhood is related to maternal diet in pregnancy. *Osteoporos Int*. 2005 Dec;16(12):1731-41. PubMed PMID: 15905998. Epub 2005/05/21. eng.

13. Jones G, Riley MD, Dwyer T. Maternal diet during pregnancy is associated with bone mineral density in children: A longitudinal study. *Eur J Clin Nutr*. 2000 Oct;54(10):749-56. PubMed PMID: 11083482. Epub 2000/11/18. eng.

14. Yin J, Dwyer T, Riley M, Cochrane J, Jones G. The association between maternal diet during pregnancy and bone mass of the children at age 16. *Eur J Clin Nutr*. 2010 Feb;64(2):131-7. PubMed PMID: 19756026. Epub 2009/09/17. eng.

15. Jarjou LM, Sawo Y, Goldberg GR, Laskey MA, Cole TJ, Prentice A. Unexpected long-term effects of calcium supplementation in pregnancy on maternal bone outcomes in women with a low calcium intake: A follow-up study. *Am J Clin Nutr*. 2013 Sep;98(3):723-30. PubMed PMID: 23902782. PubMed Central PMCID: PMC3743734. Epub 2013/08/02. eng.

16. Koo WW, Walters JC, Esterlitz J, Levine RJ, Bush AJ, Sibai B. Maternal calcium supplementation and fetal bone mineralization. *Obstet Gynecol*. 1999;94(4):577-82.

17. Raman L, Rajalakshmi K, Krishnamachari KA, Sastry JG. Effect of calcium supplementation to undernourished mothers during pregnancy on the bone density of the bone density of the neonates. *Am J Clin Nutr*. 1978 Mar;31(3):466-9. PubMed PMID: 629218. Epub 1978/03/01. eng.

18. Jarjou LM, Prentice A, Sawo Y, Laskey MA, Bennett J, Goldberg GR, et al. Randomized, placebo-controlled, calcium supplementation study in pregnant Gambian women: Effects on breast-milk calcium concentrations and infant birth weight, growth, and bone mineral accretion in the first year of life. *Am J Clin Nutr*. 2006 Mar;83(3):657-66. PubMed PMID: 16522914. Epub 2006/03/09. eng.

19. Clark EM, Ness AR, Bishop NJ, Tobias JH. Association between bone mass and fractures in children: A prospective cohort study. *J Bone Miner Res*. 2006;21(9):1489-95.

20. Harvey N, Dhanwal D, Robinson S, Kim M, Inskip H, Godfrey K, et al. Does maternal long chain polyunsaturated fatty acid status in pregnancy influence the bone health of children? The Southampton Women's Survey. *Osteoporos Int.* 2012 Sep;23(9):2359-67. PubMed PMID: 22159749. PubMed Central PMCID: Pmc3679517. Epub 2011/12/14. eng.

21. Handel MN, Moon RJ, Titcombe P, Abrahamsen B, Heitmann BL, Calder PC, et al. Maternal serum retinol and beta-carotene concentrations and neonatal bone mineralization: Results from the Southampton Women's Survey cohort. *Am J Clin Nutr.* 2016 Oct;104(4):1183-8. PubMed PMID: 27629051. Epub 2016/09/16. eng.

22. Wu AM, Huang CQ, Lin ZK, Tian NF, Ni WF, Wang XY, et al. The relationship between vitamin a and risk of fracture: Meta-analysis of prospective studies. *J Bone Miner Res.* 2014 Sep;29(9):2032-9. PubMed PMID: 24700407. Epub 2014/04/05. eng.

23. Jauniaux E, Burton GJ. Morphological and biological effects of maternal exposure to tobacco smoke on the feto-placental unit. *Early Hum Devel.* 2007;83(11):699-706.

24. Kanis JA, Johnell O, Oden A, Johansson H, De Laet C, Eisman JA, et al. Smoking and fracture risk: A meta-analysis. *Osteoporos Int.* 2005 Feb;16(2):155-62. PubMed PMID: 15175845. Epub 2004/06/04. eng.

25. Godfrey K, Walker-Bone K, Robinson S, Taylor P, Shore S, Wheeler T, et al. Neonatal bone mass: Influence of parental birthweight, maternal smoking, body composition, and activity during pregnancy. *J Bone Miner Res.* 2001 Sep;16(9):1694-703. PubMed PMID: 11547840. Epub 2001/09/08. eng.

26. Harvey NC, Javaid MK, Arden NK, Poole JR, Crozier SR, Robinson SM, et al. Maternal predictors of neonatal bone size and geometry: The Southampton Women's Survey. *J Dev Orig Health Dis.* 2010 Feb;1(1):35-41. PubMed PMID: 23750315. PubMed Central PMCID: Pmc3672833. Epub 2010/02/01. eng.

27. Martinez-Mesa J, Menezes AM, Howe LD, Wehrmeister FC, Muniz LC, Gonzalez-Chica DA, et al. Lifecourse relationship between maternal smoking during pregnancy, birth weight, contemporaneous anthropometric measurements and bone mass at 18 years old. The 1993 Pelotas Birth Cohort. *Early Hum Devel.* 2014 Dec;90(12):901-6. PubMed PMID: 25463840. PubMed Central PMCID: Pmc4252063. Epub 2014/12/03. eng.

28. Jones G, Riley M, Dwyer T. Maternal smoking during pregnancy, growth, and bone mass in prepubertal children. *J Bone Miner Res.* 1999;14(1):146-51.

29. Heppe DH, Medina-Gomez C, Hofman A, Rivadeneira F, Jaddoe VW. Does fetal smoke exposure affect childhood bone mass? The Generation R Study. *Osteoporos Int.* 2015 Apr;26(4):1319-29. PubMed PMID: 25572050. Epub 2015/01/13. eng.

30. Jones G, Hynes KL, Dwyer T. The association between breastfeeding, maternal smoking in utero, and birth weight with bone mass and fractures in adolescents: A 16-year longitudinal study. *Osteoporos Int.* 2013 May;24(5):1605-11. PubMed PMID: 23149649. Epub 2012/11/15. eng.

31. Compston JE, Flahive J, Hosmer DW, Watts NB, Siris ES, Silverman S, et al. Relationship of weight, height, and body mass index with fracture risk at different sites in postmenopausal women: The Global Longitudinal study of Osteoporosis in Women (GLOW). *J Bone Miner Res.* 2014 Feb;29(2):487-93. PubMed PMID: 23873741. Epub 2013/07/23. eng.
32. Rudang R, Mellstrom D, Clark E, Ohlsson C, Lorentzon M. Advancing maternal age is associated with lower bone mineral density in young adult male offspring. *Osteoporos Int.* 2012 Feb;23(2):475-82. PubMed PMID: 21350896. PubMed Central PMCID: Pmc3261413. Epub 2011/02/26. eng.

5

Vitamin D in early life: From observation to intervention

NICHOLAS C HARVEY, REBECCA J MOON
AND CYRUS COOPER

INTRODUCTION

There is increasing recognition that the in utero environment can modify fetal bone development with persisting effects into late childhood. Given the importance to postnatal bone mineralisation, the role of vitamin D in the fetal programming of bone development has received much interest, and the results of studies that have investigated this are discussed here.

VITAMIN D METABOLISM AND ACTIONS

Vitamin D is a secosteroid with classical functions in calcium and phosphate homeostasis. It can be derived from the diet as ergocalciferol (vitamin D_2) or cholecalciferol (vitamin D_3), or formed endogenously by the action of ultraviolet B (UVB) to convert 7-dehydrocholesterol to pre-vitamin D_3 within the skin. These pro-hormones are hydroxylated within the liver to form 25-hydroxyvitamin D [25(OH)D], which is the predominant circulating form of vitamin D. 25(OH)D acts as a reservoir for conversion to the active metabolite 1,25-dihydroxyvitamin D

[1,25(OH)$_2$D]. The main action of 1,25(OH)$_2$D is to increase the uptake of dietary calcium through increased expression of calcium transporters within the intestinal enterocytes, but it also increases production of fibroblast growth factor 23 (FGF-23), which results in phosphate wasting. Insufficient levels of vitamin D can thus result in low intestinal calcium absorption, low serum ionised calcium (Ca^{2+}) with subsequent secondary hyperparathyroidism and mobilisation of bone mineral to prevent hypocalcaemia.

Rickets and osteomalacia are the clinical endpoints of prolonged vitamin D deficiency (VDD). Rickets is a disorder of growth plate ossification and mineralisation, which only occurs in growing bone. Following fusion of the growth plates VDD can result in osteomalacia, in which the protein matrix of bone is undermineralised.

VITAMIN D DEFICIENCY IN PREGNANCY

VDD in pregnancy is common; approximately two-thirds of women in a recent study had 25(OH)D < 50 nmol/L (typically used as the definition for VDD [1]) in early and late pregnancy (2). Furthermore, at latitudes far from the equator there is marked seasonal variation in the prevalence of VDD (3), and women with darker skin pigmentation, those who use extensive skin covering for religious or cultural reasons, those who have higher body mass index (BMI), those who are younger and those who smoke are at increased risk of low 25(OH)D in pregnancy (4–7).

25(OH)D readily crosses the placenta and is the only source of 25(OH)D for the developing fetus. Thus, maternal VDD is likely to result in low levels of 25(OH)D within the fetal circulation. Indeed, maternal and umbilical cord venous blood 25(OH)D are moderately to highly correlated (8,9). Clinically, severe maternal VDD can result in neonatal hypocalcaemia causing seizures (10), and there is consistent evidence that the incidence of symptomatic neonatal hypocalcaemia can be reduced by antenatal vitamin D supplementation (11–13). Cases of infants with early-onset rickets, including the classical bony abnormalities, have also been reported, but these children are typically born to mothers with severe VDD, clinical signs of osteomalacia and originating from populations at high risk of VDD and/or received limited antenatal care (14). However, there is now increasing evidence that maternal vitamin D supplementation might be of benefit to prenatal bone development in the wider population.

PRENATAL VITAMIN D EXPOSURE AND BONE DEVELOPMENT: OBSERVATIONAL DATA

Some of the earliest data to suggest that vitamin D exposure might influence in utero bone mineral accrual used season as a proxy marker of vitamin D status. Namgung et al. found that in 71 Korean neonates, those born in summer (July–December) had 8% higher whole body (WB) bone mineral content (BMC) after adjustment for weight than infants born in winter (January–March). Furthermore, in this cohort, neonatal 25(OH)D measured at delivery was positively correlated with WB BMC (15). In contrast, the same authors found that infants in the United States born in the summer months had lower WB BMC than winter-born infants (16). The authors proposed that these differences reflect the use of vitamin D supplementation in the two populations; the uptake of supplementation is low throughout pregnancy in Korea but standard practice after the first trimester in the United States, where differences in maternal 25(OH)D by season of birth were not observed (15). As such, this would suggest that early pregnancy 25(OH)D status might be important for fetal bone mineralisation.

Subsequent studies have used measurements of maternal or cord blood 25(OH)D. Weiler et al. studied 50 neonates born in Canada between April and August. 25(OH)D was measured in venous cord blood and used to divide the infants into two groups using a cut point of 37.5 nmol/L. The infants in the low 25(OH)D group tended to be heavier and longer, but this might have reflected the greater ethnic diversity in the group compared to the high 25(OH)D group. However, WB and femur BMC relative to body weight were significantly lower in the 18 neonates with a cord blood 25(OH)D < 37.5 nmol/L compared with 32 infants with a 25(OH)D above this cut-point (17). Similarly, Viljakainen et al., using the mean of two maternal serum 25(OH)D measurements from early pregnancy and 2 days postpartum as the assessment of maternal vitamin D status, found neonatal tibial BMC and cross-sectional area (CSA) measured by peripheral quantitative computed tomography (pQCT) were 14% and 16% higher, respectively, in 98 infants born to mothers with 25(OH)D above the median for the cohort. Although volumetric bone mineral density (BMD) of the tibia did not differ between the two groups, the difference in BMC and CSA did persist after adjustment for weight (18). When a subset of these children was reassessed at 14 months of age, the difference in tibial BMC was no longer present, but tibial CSA remained significantly higher in those born to mothers with higher vitamin D status in pregnancy (Figure 5.1) (19). Conversely, in 125 Gambian mother-offspring pairs, no significant relationships were observed between maternal 25(OH)D at either 20 or 36 weeks gestation and offspring whole-body BMC or bone area at 2, 13 or 52 weeks of age (20). In contrast to the other studies, none of the mothers had a 25(OH)D below 50 nmol/L, which is consistent with the notion that poorer skeletal mineralisation might only occur in fetuses of mothers with the lowest vitamin D levels.

There is some evidence to suggest that these relationships persist into childhood, although study findings are less consistent than in the neonatal period. Positive relationships between maternal 25(OH)D measured in late pregnancy and offspring whole-body and lumbar spine bone area, BMC and areal BMD (aBMD) at 9 years of age in 198 mother-offspring pairs in the Princess Anne Hospital Study (Southampton, UK) were reported by Javaid et al. (Figure 5.2) (21). Beneficial effects of vitamin D supplementation were also suggested by this study as children born to women who consumed vitamin D–containing supplements had higher whole-body BMC and bone area, but not aBMD. Although the women who took supplements were self-selected, this finding was not changed by adjustment for socioeconomic status. Positive associations were also observed between maternal 25(OH)D and umbilical venous calcium concentration, suggesting the effect of vitamin D on skeletal development might be mediated through placental calcium transport.

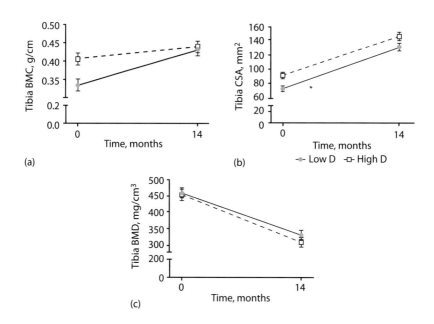

Figure 5.1 Offspring BMC (a), CSA (b) and BMD (c) in study groups from baseline to 14 months. Low D and High D groups are represented by circles and squares, respectively. Error bars represent standard error of mean (SEM). (Reproduced with permission from Viljakainen HT et al. *Osteoporos Int.* 2011 Mar;22(3):883-91.)

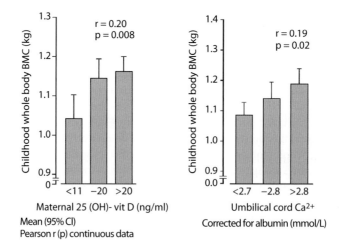

Figure 5.2 Maternal 25(OH)D in late pregnancy and offspring bone mass at 9 years. (Based on data from Javaid MK et al. *Lancet.* 2006;367(9504):36-43.)

These findings were replicated in a larger cohort, the Southampton Women's Survey (SWS), at the same research centre, in which 1030 mother-offspring pairs had measurement of 25(OH)D at 34 weeks' gestation and whole body less head (WBLH) and lumbar spine DXA at 6 to 7 years. WBLH BMC, bone area, BMD and lumbar spine BMC were all significantly lower in children born to mothers with 25(OH)D < 25 nmol/L in late pregnancy, including after adjustment for maternal age, ethnicity, height, prepregnancy BMI, smoking in late pregnancy, social class, maternal educational attainment and duration of breast feeding (22). Similarly, the Raine cohort in Western Australia also found a positive relationship between maternal vitamin D status at 18 weeks' gestation and peak bone mass. Thus after adjustment for sex, age, height and body composition at age 20 years, maternal height and prepregnancy weight, maternal age at delivery, parity, education, ethnicity, smoking during pregnancy and season of maternal blood sampling, WB BMC and aBMD were 2.7% and 1.7% lower at 20 years of age in offspring of mothers with 25(OH)D < 50 nmol/L compared to those above this level (23).

In contrast, findings from the Avon Longitudinal Study of Parents and Children (ALSPAC), a large mother-offspring cohort study in the Avon region, UK, do not support these studies. Initially, using 6995 mother-offspring pairs, a positive relationship was found between estimated maternal UVB exposure in late pregnancy used as a proxy marker for 25(OH)D and offspring WBLH BMC, bone area and BMD at 9.9 years of age (24). However, further analysis in a subset of 3960 of the children for whom maternal serum 25(OH)D measurement was available in the first (n = 1035), second (n = 879) or third (n = 2046) trimester did not reveal any significant associations between maternal 25(OH)D and offspring bone mineralisation (25). The authors suggest that collinearity of the estimated maternal UVB measurement with age at DXA assessment (an unexpected quirk in the original dataset) confounded the relationships in the initial study. Nonetheless, these findings highlight the need for high quality intervention studies.

INTERVENTION STUDIES OF ANTENATAL VITAMIN D SUPPLEMENTATION AND OFFSPRING BONE DEVELOPMENT

The first study to assess the effect of antenatal vitamin D supplementation on offspring bone mineralisation was undertaken by Congdon et al. and published in 1983. Sixty-four women of Asian ethnicity living in the United Kingdom participated in a non-randomised study; 19 received a daily supplement containing 1000 IU vitamin D and calcium (of unknown strength) during the last trimester, whereas 45 received no supplementation. There was no significant difference in forearm BMC of the offspring at birth assessed using single photon absorptiometry (26), but the study size, lack of randomisation and technology used limits the interpretation of the findings.

There are three more recently published studies of gestational vitamin D supplementation, of which the largest is the Maternal Vitamin D Osteoporosis Study

(MAVIDOS). The primary outcome of MAVIDOS, a randomised double-blind placebo-controlled trial of antenatal vitamin D supplementation from 14 weeks' gestation until delivery conducted over three centres in the UK, was neonatal bone mass (27). Eleven hundred thirty-four women with a baseline 25(OH)D between 25 and 100 nmol/L were randomised to 1000 IU/day cholecalciferol or placebo. Nine hundred sixty-five remained in the study until delivery, and 736 infants had WB and lumbar spine DXA. Although there were no differences in WB or LS BMC, bone area or aBMD between the two groups overall, in a pre-specified analysis, there was a statistically significant interaction between season of birth and treatment (Figure 5.3) (2).

Thus, WB BMC and BMD were approximately 9% and 5% higher, respectively, in the children born in winter to mothers randomised to cholecalciferol compared to those randomised to placebo, the differences being highly statistically significant (p = 0.004 for BMC). This effect size is substantially larger than those observed between children with and without fractures (28), being, for BMC, equivalent to around a 0.5 standard deviation (SD) difference, and hence if persisting into later childhood are likely to be clinically relevant.

These findings would support the notion that the last trimester is the critical window for fetal bone mineral accretion (indeed the majority of the calcium

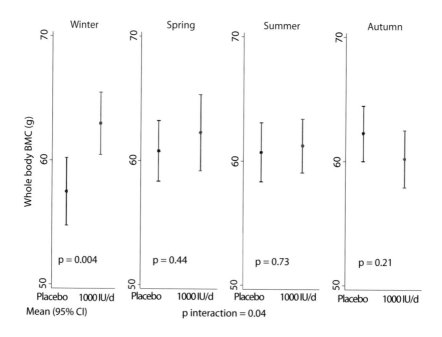

Figure 5.3 Neonatal whole body bone mineral content (BMC) by intervention group and season of birth. Data shown are mean and 95% CI. Winter is December to February, spring is March to May, summer is June to August, and autumn is September to November. (Adapted from Cooper C et al. *Lancet Diabetes Endocrinol.* 2016 May;4(5):393-402.)

required for fetal skeletal mineralisation is transferred from mother to fetus in these later stages of pregnancy), and although supplementation with 1000 IU/day did not result in the same achieved 25(OH)D in women who delivered in winter compared to summer months, supplementation did prevent the decline in 25(OH)D status from early to late pregnancy observed in mothers who delivered in winter and were randomised to placebo (2) (Figure 5.4). Consistent with these results, similar findings come from the SWS, in which summer/autumn births had higher neonatal BMC than did winter/spring births (63 g vs 61 g; p = 0.03, Figure 5.5).

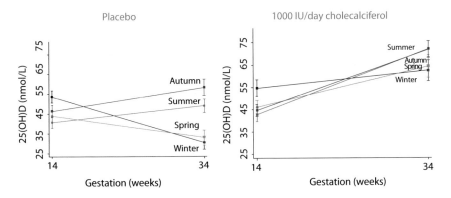

Figure 5.4 Maternal 25(OH)D status at baseline (14 weeks' gestation) and 34 weeks' gestation by intervention group and season of birth. Data shown are mean and 95% confidence interval. Winter is December to February, spring is March to May, summer is June to August and autumn is September to November. (Adapted from Cooper C et al. *Lancet Diabetes Endocrinol.* 2016 May;4(5):393-402.)

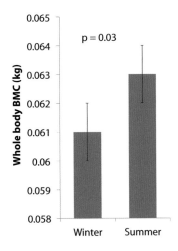

Figure 5.5 Season of birth and neonatal whole body bone mineral content (BMC) in the Southampton Women's Survey. Summer is June to November, winter is December to May. Data are mean and 95% confidence interval.

Two small intervention studies from India and Iran have also assessed bone mass in infants born to mothers randomised to vitamin D supplementation or placebo. Sahoo et al. randomised 300 women to three groups which received 400 IU/day cholecalciferol daily ('placebo'), 60,000 IU cholecalciferol every 4 weeks or 60,000 IU cholecalciferol every 8 weeks from the second trimester. All women also received daily calcium supplementation. Only 160 women were followed up until delivery, and 52 children (17% of the original cohort) underwent DXA at 12 to 16 months. The children in the placebo group were significantly older at DXA scan and had higher measurements of WB BMC and BMD, but in multivariate analysis randomisation group was not a significant predictor of BMC or BMD (29). Vaziri et al. randomised 153 women to placebo or 2000 IU/day cholecalciferol from 26 to 28 weeks until delivery, but only 25 infants (16% of the cohort) had DXA assessment. No significant difference in WB BMC, BMD or BA was found (30), but as with the study by Sahoo et al., the small numbers included are unlikely to have sufficient power to detect a difference in the outcomes studied.

CONCLUSION

Evidence from observational studies does suggest that achieving higher levels of serum 25(OH)D in pregnancy might have beneficial effects on offspring bone development. Recent findings from the MAVIDOS study would suggest that supplementation of those pregnant women who are due to deliver infants in winter months with 1000 IU/day from the start of the second trimester will increase the bone mass of the offspring in the neonatal period. However, replication of this finding in other large studies and further follow-up into later childhood (both of which are currently ongoing) to ensure the positive effects on bone mineralisation persist is required before this finding can be confidently translated into public health advice.

REFERENCES

1. Ross AC, Manson JE, Abrams SA, Aloia JF, Brannon PM, Clinton SK, et al. The 2011 report on dietary reference intakes for calcium and vitamin D from the Institute of Medicine: What clinicians need to know. *J Clin Endocrinol Metab.* 2011 Jan;96(1):53-8. PubMed PMID: 21118827. PubMed Central PMCID: PMC3046611. Epub 2010/12/02. eng.
2. Cooper C, Harvey NC, Bishop NJ, Kennedy S, Papageorghiou AT, Schoenmakers I, et al. Maternal gestational vitamin D supplementation and offspring bone health (MAVIDOS): A multicentre, double-blind, randomised placebo-controlled trial. *Lancet Diabetes Endocrinol.* 2016 May;4(5):393-402. PubMed PMID: 26944421. PubMed Central PMCID: PMC4843969. Epub 2016/03/06. eng.

3. Moon RJ, Crozier SR, Dennison EM, Davies JH, Robinson SM, Inskip HM, et al. Tracking of 25-hydroxyvitamin D status during pregnancy: The importance of vitamin D supplementation. *Am J Clin Nutr.* 2015 Nov; 102(5):1081-7. PubMed PMID: 26399867. PubMed Central PMCID: PMC4634223. Epub 2015/09/25. eng.

4. Crozier SR, Harvey NC, Inskip HM, Godfrey KM, Cooper C, Robinson SM. Maternal vitamin D status in pregnancy is associated with adiposity in the offspring: Findings from the Southampton Women's Survey. *Am J Clin Nutr.* 2012 7/2012;96(1):57-63.

5. Andersen LB, Abrahamsen B, Dalgard C, Kyhl HB, Beck-Nielsen SS, Frost-Nielsen M, et al. Parity and tanned white skin as novel predictors of vitamin D status in early pregnancy: A population-based cohort study. *Clin Endocrinol (Oxf).* 2013 Sep;79(3):333-41. PubMed PMID: 23305099. Epub 2013/01/12. eng.

6. Schneuer FJ, Roberts CL, Guilbert C, Simpson JM, Algert CS, Khambalia AZ, et al. Effects of maternal serum 25-hydroxyvitamin D concentrations in the first trimester on subsequent pregnancy outcomes in an Australian population. *Am J Clin Nutr.* 2014 Feb;99(2):287-95. PubMed PMID: 24257720. Epub 2013/11/22. eng.

7. Xiao JP, Zang J, Pei JJ, Xu F, Zhu Y, Liao XP. Low maternal vitamin D status during the second trimester of pregnancy: A cross-sectional study in Wuxi, China. *PloS One.* 2015;10(2):e0117748. PubMed PMID: 25659105. PubMed Central PMCID: Pmc4320063. Epub 2015/02/07. eng.

8. Grant CC, Stewart AW, Scragg R, Milne T, Rowden J, Ekeroma A, et al. Vitamin D during pregnancy and infancy and infant serum 25-hydroxyvitamin D concentration. *Pediatrics.* 2013 Dec 16. PubMed PMID: 24344104. Epub 2013/12/18. eng.

9. Song SJ, Si S, Liu J, Chen X, Zhou L, Jia G, et al. Vitamin D status in Chinese pregnant women and their newborns in Beijing and their relationships to birth size. *Public Health Nutr.* 2013 Apr;16(4):687-92. PubMed PMID: 23174124. Epub 2012/11/24. eng.

10. Erdeve O, Atasay B, Arsan S, Siklar Z, Ocal G, Berberoglu M. Hypocalcemic seizure due to congenital rickets in the first day of life. *Turkish J Pediatr.* 2007 Jul-Sep;49(3):301-3. PubMed PMID: 17990585. Epub 2007/11/10. eng.

11. Brooke OG, Brown IR, Bone CD, Carter ND, Cleeve HJ, Maxwell JD, et al. Vitamin D supplements in pregnant Asian women: Effects on calcium status and fetal growth. *BMJ.* 1980 Mar 15;280(6216):751-4. PubMed PMID: 6989438. PubMed Central PMCID: Pmc1600591. Epub 1980/03/15. eng.

12. Cockburn F, Belton NR, Purvis RJ, Giles MM, Brown JK, Turner TL, et al. Maternal vitamin D intake and mineral metabolism in mothers and their newborn infants. *BMJ.* 1980 Jul 5;281(6232):11-4. PubMed PMID: 7407476. PubMed Central PMCID: Pmc1713762. Epub 1980/07/05. eng.

13. Hashemipour S, Lalooha F, Zahir Mirdamadi S, Ziaee A, Dabaghi Ghaleh T. Effect of vitamin D administration in vitamin D-deficient pregnant women on maternal and neonatal serum calcium and vitamin D concentrations: A randomised clinical trial. *Br J Nutr.* 2013 Nov 14;110(9):1611-6. PubMed PMID: 23628132. Epub 2013/05/01. eng.

14. Elidrissy AT. The return of congenital rickets, are we missing occult cases? *Calcif Tissue Int.* 2016 Sep;99(3):227-36. PubMed PMID: 27245342. Epub 2016/06/02. eng.

15. Namgung R, Tsang RC, Lee C, Han DG, Ho ML, Sierra RI. Low total body bone mineral content and high bone resorption in Korean winter-born versus summer-born newborn infants. *J Pediatr.* 1998 3/1998;132(3 Pt 1):421-5.

16. Namgung R, Tsang RC. Factors affecting newborn bone mineral content: In utero effects on newborn bone mineralization. *Proc Nutr Soc.* 2000; 59(1):55-63.

17. Weiler H, Fitzpatrick-Wong S, Veitch R, Kovacs H, Schellenberg J, McCloy U, et al. Vitamin D deficiency and whole-body and femur bone mass relative to weight in healthy newborns. *CMAJ.* 2005 3/15/2005;172(6):757-61.

18. Viljakainen HT, Saarnio E, Hytinantti T, Miettinen M, Surcel H, Makitie O, et al. Maternal vitamin D status determines bone variables in the newborn. *J Clin Endocrinol Metab.* 2010 Apr;95(4):1749-57. PubMed PMID: 20139235.

19. Viljakainen HT, Korhonen T, Hytinantti T, Laitinen EK, Andersson S, Makitie O, et al. Maternal vitamin D status affects bone growth in early childhood – A prospective cohort study. *Osteoporos Int.* 2011 Mar;22(3):883-91. PubMed PMID: 21153404. PubMed Central PMCID: 3034879.

20. Prentice A, Jarjou LM, Goldberg GR, Bennett J, Cole TJ, Schoenmakers I. Maternal plasma 25-hydroxyvitamin D concentration and birthweight, growth and bone mineral accretion of Gambian infants. *Acta Paediatr.* 2009 Aug;98(8):1360-2. PubMed PMID: 19594476. PubMed Central PMCID: PMC2721965. Epub 2009/07/15. eng.

21. Javaid MK, Crozier SR, Harvey NC, Gale CR, Dennison EM, Boucher BJ, et al. Maternal vitamin D status during pregnancy and childhood bone mass at age 9 years: A longitudinal study. *Lancet.* 2006;367(9504):36-43.

22. Moon RJ, Harvey NC, Davies JH, Cooper C. Vitamin D and bone development. *Osteoporos Int.* 2015 Apr;26(4):1449-51. PubMed PMID: 25448839. Epub 2014/12/03. eng.

23. Zhu K, Whitehouse AJ, Hart P, Kusel M, Mountain J, Lye S, et al. Maternal Vitamin D Status During Pregnancy and Bone Mass in Offspring at 20 Years of Age: A Prospective Cohort Study. *J Bone Miner Res.* 2013 Nov 5. PubMed PMID: 24189972. Epub 2013/11/06. eng.

24. Sayers A, Tobias JH. Estimated maternal ultraviolet B exposure levels in pregnancy influence skeletal development of the child. *J Clin Endocrinol Metab.* 2009 Mar;94(3):765-71. PubMed PMID: 19116232. PubMed Central PMCID: 2742727.

25. Lawlor DA, Wills AK, Fraser A, Sayers A, Fraser WD, Tobias JH. Association of maternal vitamin D status during pregnancy with bone-mineral content in offspring: A prospective cohort study. *Lancet.* 2013;381(9884):2176-83.

26. Congdon P, Horsman A, Kirby PA, Dibble J, Bashir T. Mineral content of the forearms of babies born to Asian and white mothers. *BMJ (Clin Res Ed).* 1983 Apr 16;286(6373):1233-5. PubMed PMID: 6404403. PubMed Central PMCID: Pmc1547285. Epub 1983/04/16. eng.

27. Harvey NC, Javaid K, Bishop N, Kennedy S, Papageorghiou AT, Fraser R, et al. MAVIDOS Maternal Vitamin D Osteoporosis Study: Study protocol for a randomized controlled trial. The MAVIDOS Study Group. *Trials.* 2012 2012;13:13.

28. Clark EM, Ness AR, Bishop NJ, Tobias JH. Association between bone mass and fractures in children: A prospective cohort study. *J Bone Miner Res.* 2006;21(9):1489-95.

29. Sahoo SK, Katam KK, Das V, Agarwal A, Bhatia V. Maternal vitamin D supplementation in pregnancy and offspring outcomes: A double-blind randomized placebo-controlled trial. *J Bone Miner Metab.* 2016 Sep 14. PubMed PMID: 27628045. Epub 2016/09/16. eng.

30. Vaziri F, Dabbaghmanesh MH, Samsami A, Nasiri S, Shirazi PT. Vitamin D supplementation during pregnancy on infant anthropometric measurements and bone mass of mother-infant pairs: A randomized placebo clinical trial. *Early Hum Dev.* 2016 Aug 8;103:61-8. PubMed PMID: 27513714. Epub 2016/08/12. eng.

6

Nutrition and bone health during childhood and adolescence: A global perspective

KATE A WARD, ANN PRENTICE, SHANE A NORRIS
AND JOHN M PETTIFOR

INTRODUCTION

Charles Dent described senile osteoporosis as a paediatric disease, and over the past two decades the understanding of the importance of the growing years to future musculoskeletal health has increased, highlighting the importance of taking a lifecourse approach for prevention of disease. By 2050, 2 billion of the global population will be aged over 60 years, and the vast majority of the ageing population will live in low- and middle-income countries (LMIC) (1). It is predicted that the rise in the ageing population in LMIC will be associated with a concomitant rise in noncommunicable disease risk, and this includes osteoporosis and other musculoskeletal diseases (2,3). To date there is limited knowledge within these countries of the importance of diet and nutrition to skeletal growth and health.

Skeletal growth is a composite term for growth in length (increase in height), growth in width (increase in cross-section) and the accrual of mineral (mainly calcium, phosphorus and magnesium) into the collagen framework of the bone. During growth, there is constant modelling and remodelling of bones to adapt size, shape and mineral content to ensure they remain fit-for-purpose and do not fracture under normal daily loading. As longitudinal growth ceases and skeletal maturity is reached, 'peak bone mass' is attained, which creates the reservoir of bone mineral for later life (Figure 6.1). Whilst traditionally peak bone mass is envisaged as the amount of mineral within the skeleton, by the end of growth, the shape, size and distribution of bone tissue within the periosteal envelope have been determined, all of which are important contributors to the strength of a bone. After that time there is no net gain of bone mineral, just remodelling to repair and replace old bone tissue, small increases in bone size and changes in distribution to maintain strength as efficiently as possible. The capacity of an individual to reach peak bone mass that is not lower than their genetic potential is dependent on internal and external environmental factors (4). Internal environment describes innate factors, such as genotype and consequent phenotype, and external environment are those factors which may illicit a physiological

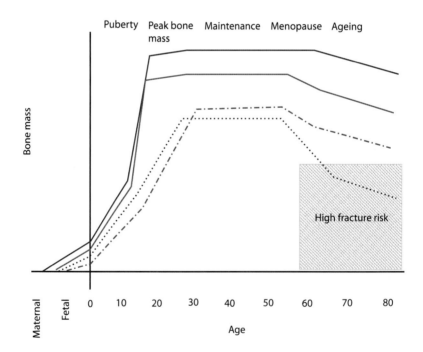

Figure 6.1 Trajectories of bone accrual and loss though life and potential consequences for fracture risk. The blue solid line is males; pink solid line, females; grey dotted line, populations with delayed puberty not currently at high fracture risk; black dotted line, individuals from populations where slower and poorer growth is a risk factor for higher fracture risk.

response and are modifiable such as birth size, diet and physical activity (4,5). Disentangling the effects of all of these factors is clearly complex, as many are inter-related. By using the available longitudinal data from cohorts and trials from across the globe it is possible to investigate how growth affects future bone health and fracture risk. These data now include countries where the ageing population is rising fastest, such as South Africa and India. It is also possible to identify those external factors that can be modified during growth to optimise bone health and to prevent the predicted rise in fracture rates in LMIC (3,6).

In this chapter, the focus is on how diet and nutrition influence future bone health, firstly by describing relationships between later fracture risk and growth in childhood and adolescence, and then by describing the current state of knowledge of nutritional rickets across the globe. Before that, it is necessary to briefly consider how the growing skeleton may be quantitatively assessed.

SKELETAL ASSESSMENT DURING GROWTH

Bone mass (g) is, by definition, the amount of mineral contained within a volume of bone (usually the whole skeleton) and is derived from volumetric bone mineral density (vBMD) and bone volume. Dual-energy X-ray absorptiometry (DXA) is the gold standard measurement used clinically and in the majority of paediatric research. DXA-derived measures of areal bone mineral density (aBMD, g/cm^2) or bone mineral content (BMC, g) are used as surrogates of bone strength for assessment of bone health. DXA has limitations because it estimates an aBMD, not vBMD, from a two-dimensional image and therefore does not take into account the depth of a bone. aBMD only partially adjusts for bone size differences and is therefore an overestimation of vBMD in larger children and an underestimation in small children; this size artefact also therefore affects longitudinal measurements during growth. Size-adjustment of DXA measures is therefore imperative, and several methods are available (7–14): (i) calculation of an apparent volumetric density (bone mineral apparent density [BMAD]), by assuming the vertebrae are cuboid or cylindrical in shape (7,10); (ii) use of regression models to 'fully' adjust for the size component taking into account height, weight or lean mass, bone area (size-adjusted BMC [SA-BMC]) (8,9,11); (iii) use of size-adjusted prediction equations using height-for-age z-scores and (iv) the 'Molgaard' three-step approach assessing whether bones are short for age (height for age), narrow for height (bone area for height) and 'light' for size (BMC for bone area) (13). To date, there is insufficient evidence as to which of these is the best predictor of fracture in either healthy children or those with acute or chronic disease, but there is consensus that DXA-measures of aBMD or BMC should be interpreted taking a child's size and maturation into account, and definitely not used in isolation (15,16). In addition, studies investigating determinants of bone measures or changes over time are especially affected if size-adjustment is not carried out when the variables of interest are also related to the size of the individual.

The use of quantitative methods that are less size dependent and that measure a volume of bone, making assessment of vBMD possible, is increasing, particularly in research. Peripheral quantitative computed tomography (pQCT), whether single-slice or more recently high resolution (see Chapter 11), is the most commonly used method (17). Peripheral and high-resolution pQCT are advantageous as they measure other important aspects of bone strength, including separate measures of the cortical and trabecular compartments, and provide assessments of microarchitecture and strength with good precision and with as low ionising radiation exposure as DXA (18). Central QCT is also used, but less frequently due to its greater ionising radiation exposure and lack of accessibility to scanners.

CHILDHOOD AND ADOLESCENT GROWTH, AND ADULT FRACTURE RISK

Figure 6.1 illustrates the accrual of bone during growth. It is clear from this that the childhood and adolescent growth period is crucial for future bone health; 30% to 40% of bone mass is accrued during the pubertal growth spurt (19,20). Chapter 3 discusses the association between early growth and fracture risk. Evidence also exists of the importance of later childhood and adolescent growth on adult bone outcomes and on fracture risk. The epidemiology of childhood growth and future fracture risk was described in two Finnish cohorts where birth records and childhood growth were linked to hospital discharge records (21–23). A low rate of height and weight growth, and in BMI accrual, was associated with increased risk of adult hip fracture. More recently, data from prospective birth cohorts with long-term health outcomes, such as the MRC National Survey for Health and Development, have made it possible to study in more detail growth, pubertal timing and consequences for musculoskeletal ageing (24–27). Bone length, width and BMD were related to the timing of peak height velocity in adulthood (24,25). Weight gain during puberty was associated with vBMD and aBMD (24). From these studies, we can conclude that changes in environment, whether natural or via interventions that impact the timing of puberty or the speed at which growth proceeds and weight is gained, may alter attainment of final height and peak bone mass (mineral content and skeletal size).

Far fewer data are available from LMIC, where the projected rise in fracture incidence is greatest. In the New Delhi cohort, similar results to those above were found. Greater height gain in infancy, and BMI gain during childhood and adolescence were positively associated with BMC, aBMD and BMAD (28). When adult height and BMI were corrected for, the associations were attenuated, showing this was an association with growth rather than bone mineralisation.

NUTRITION AND GROWTH

Diet and nutrition influence bone growth through multiple and interrelated, pathways: (i) provision of minerals required for bone formation (calcium, phosphorus, magnesium), and of those involved more generally in growth and the timing of puberty (e.g. zinc, copper, iron); (ii) supply of vitamins involved in calcium-phosphate homeostasis (e.g. vitamins D and K); (iii) supply of energy, amino acids and ions; (iv) their role in the development of muscle strength; (v) being under- or overweight, which determines skeletal loading; and (vi) through influence on the timing of pubertal growth where delay and advancement are related to under- and overnutrition, respectively (4,18,29). The majority of the evidence with regard to bone health comes from cross-sectional associations between calcium intake, 25(OH)D status and bone mineral content or density (SA-BMC, BMD) or from interventions of single nutrients such as calcium, vitamin D or protein. The focus in this chapter is on calcium and vitamin D, deficiencies of which are important in the development of nutritional rickets, as described later.

Calcium

Despite being the most abundant mineral in bone, the evidence for an association between calcium intake and bone growth/development/health is weak and inconsistent. The prospective Bone Mineral Density in Childhood Study reported weak positive associations at the lumbar spine between self-reported calcium intake and BMC accrual during growth; physical activity was more strongly and consistently associated with BMC across race and sex subgroups (30). Similarly, in a rural Indian cohort, current calcium intake and vitamin D status were not consistent predictors of aBMD at the hip and spine at age 18 to 23 years; lean mass was the strongest predictor (31). A few randomised controlled trials (RCTs) have demonstrated sustained benefits of supplementation once the intervention ceases, particularly where the supplementation was in the form of calcium salts rather than dairy derivatives (32–40). For calcium, many of the reported increases in aBMD are thought to be through a bone remodelling transient, whereby increased calcium intake temporarily lowers bone turnover rates and reduces the number of bone remodelling units. This results in an apparent increase in measured aBMD or BMC, but once calcium intakes return to pre-supplementation levels, turnover is restored and the transient increase in aBMD returns to baseline level. Other studies suggest that rather than an increase in bone mineralisation, the calcium effect is because puberty is brought forward by the supplementation, so it is the growth difference that the DXA data are reflecting rather than a net increase in aBMD or BMC (41–43). Milk protein has been associated with SA-BMC independent of IGF-1 and calcium in one study, and some, but not all, trials of dairy sources of calcium have shown a sustained increase in BMD or BMC, although, importantly, it was often not possible in these studies to include a sufficiently long follow-up period to confirm these findings (32–34,44).

Most calcium supplementation studies have been conducted in populations with adequate habitual calcium intakes, which may explain the lack of consistency in findings. It may be reasonable to expect that intervention in populations with extremely low calcium intake and/or poor vitamin D status may be more beneficial to bone and for the consequent effects to be sustained. Somewhat surprisingly, despite most studies reporting an initial increase in BMD/SA-BMC, after a period of follow-up the differences between intervention and control groups is attenuated (35,36,45–47). The longest post-supplement period of follow-up is from The Gambia, West Africa, where daily calcium intakes are on average 300 mg/day. Prepubertal children aged 8 to 11 years were given 1000 mg calcium or placebo, 5 days per week for a year (ISRCTN28836000). They were then followed to the end of growth, approximately 12 years later. At the end of the trial and after 1 and 2 years post-supplementation, the calcium group had higher SA-BMC (35,36); mean (SE) 4.6 (0.9)% reducing to 2.5 (1.3)% after 2 years follow-up. After longitudinal growth modelling of the whole period of follow-up, group differences, split by sex, in pubertal timing, the velocity of growth and final 'size' were determined (42,43). In boys who took calcium, pubertal timing (age at peak height velocity) was brought forward by approximately 7 months, and although they transitioned through puberty at the same velocity as the placebo group they stopped growing earlier (42) (Figure 6.2). As a consequence, the boys in the calcium group were taller and had greater BMC in mid-adolescence but were on average 3.5cm shorter at the end of the follow-up period. There were no significant group differences in bone outcomes at the end of growth, which may suggest that the supplementation had an effect on longitudinal growth rather than directly on bone mineralisation (43). In girls, no significant differences were found in the amount of bone accrued (BMC or BA) or in the timing of puberty; we considered that this may have been because the early stages of puberty, before physical signs become evident, were already initiated in these females prior to the start of the supplementation (42,48). The long-term consequences of these findings cannot be confirmed without further follow-up of the cohort.

Vitamin D

There have been fewer intervention trials of vitamin D supplementation in children and adolescents. The Institute of Medicine (US) and more recently the Scientific Advisory Committee for Nutrition (UK), concluded that although there were plenty of studies showing associations between 25(OH)D status and BMD, the limited evidence available from RCTs did not support a consistent benefit of supplementation on BMD in children and adolescents (49,50). The results of a meta-analysis, in which only six trials were eligible for inclusion, showed little evidence to support supplementation in children, although when stratified by baseline 25(OH)D concentration, those with lowest, arbitrarily selected baseline levels had significantly higher BMC (1.7% and 2.6%, depending on bone site) after supplementation (51). Trials in populations with low baseline 25(OH)D concentrations (25–27.5 nmol/L) have found mixed effects of the intervention on BMD. The timing of supplementation seems to be important: in a trial from Lebanon, greater changes were reported in pre-puberty and pre-menarche girls compared to a post-menarche group (52,53). A follow-up period was included, and after 12 and 24 months there were significantly greater differences in BMD and BMC in the vitamin D group, although some were attenuated after adjusting for size; hip BMC remained of borderline significance (53). No effects of supplementation were found in boys in the initial trial or at any stage of follow-up (52,53). In South Asian post-menarcheal and asymptomatic girls from the UK, significant improvements in muscle power were reported after a year's supplementation with vitamin D_2; no effects were seen on bone, but it should be noted that bone age- and sex-matched z-scores were not significantly reduced in the group

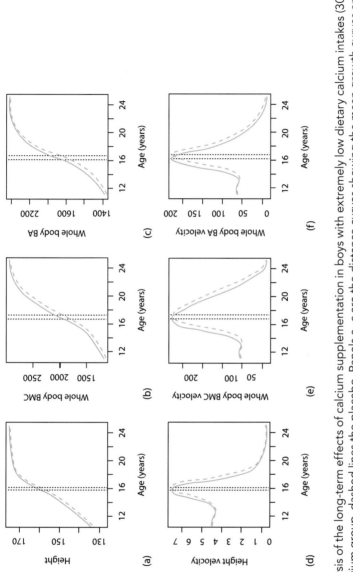

Figure 6.2 SITAR analysis of the long-term effects of calcium supplementation in boys with extremely low dietary calcium intakes (300 mg/day). Solid lines are calcium group, dashed lines the placebo. Panels a–c are the distance curves showing the mean growth curves and final height, bone mineral content and bone area of each group. Panels d–f are the velocity curves. The vertical lines on d–f show mean age of peak height velocity in each group. Puberty is brought forward in the calcium group but they stop growing earlier, and are shorter (a) at the end of growth. There were no sustained effects on bone mineral content (b) or area (c). BA, bone area; BMC, bone mineral content. (Adapted from Prentice A et al. *Am J Clin Nutr*, 2012, 96(5):1042-50 and Ward et al. *J Clin Endocrinol Metab*, 2014, 99(9):3169-76.)

at the start of the intervention despite extremely low 25(OH)D status at baseline (54). In post-menarcheal girls from India, whilst improvements in 25(OH)D status were found, there were no overall effects on bone; differences in SA-BMC and BA were found in those who were closest to menarche (55). The response to supplementation may also depend on genotype: in a trial from Denmark, girls with FF genotype for the Fok 1 polymorphism showed significant increases in whole body BMD and BMC, but in the trial overall there was no effect of supplementation. In contrast, a study from India demonstrated no association between change in BMD, SA-BMC and the Fok 1 genotype (56). Further work is needed to understand whether the effects of vitamin D supplementation are on growth, mineralisation and/or on muscle function and mass.

In summary, there is little evidence from trials or from longitudinal growth data to suggest that intervention with calcium or vitamin D has a sustained effect on bone in populations with low or suboptimal calcium intakes and/or 25(OH)D status. Nevertheless, as described below, extremely low dietary calcium intakes and 25(OH)D levels in the vitamin D–deficient range (<30 nmol/L) may lead to rickets. Where sustained differences are reported, they suggest a growth effect and require further mechanistic follow-up. Importantly, interventions may improve early growth or bone health but may have long-term unintended consequences on the trajectory of growth of an individual. There appear to be differences in response, particularly to vitamin D, depending on the stage of growth during which the intervention occurs, and this is to some extent seen also in calcium trials. This may be the reason sex differences are observed in response to supplementation. The next part of this chapter focuses on the role of calcium and vitamin D deficiency in relation to clinical manifestations of rickets, osteomalacia and associated conditions.

NUTRITION AND RICKETS IN CHILDHOOD

It was highlighted above that calcium and/or vitamin D supplementation has little effect on bone health; however, the consequence of prolonged severe deficiency of either of these two nutrients individually or in combination may be a failure of mineralisation of bone and growth plate matrix. Nutritional rickets is a public health concern in many countries globally due to the high prevalence of vitamin D and/or dietary calcium deficiency in at-risk populations. The deleterious consequences of rickets relate not only to the clinical effects during active rickets, such as those associated with perturbations of calcium homeostasis, but also to the consequences of impaired growth and deformities that develop at the growth plates, and the possible increased morbidity and mortality of lower respiratory tract infections associated with vitamin D deficiency, as well as the long-term effects of limb and pelvic deformities.

Central to the pathogenesis of nutritional rickets is the inability to maintain normocalcaemia, which may occur as a result of either impaired intestinal calcium absorption as a consequence of vitamin D deficiency, or through inadequate intestinal calcium absorption due to low dietary calcium intakes (Figure 6.3). The fall in plasma ionized calcium concentration sets up a sequence of events which

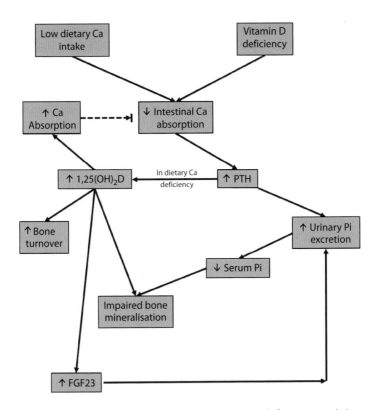

Figure 6.3 The interrelationships between vitamin D deficiency and dietary calcium deficiency in the pathogenesis of nutritional rickets.

leads to secondary hyperparathyroidism and consequent hypophosphataemia, impaired chondrocyte maturation and delayed and impaired mineralisation of the growth plate cartilage matrix and osteoid.

Vitamin D deficiency rickets (and associated osteomalacia) has a peak incidence from 6 months to about 2 years of age, with another peak occurring during the pubertal growth spurt. Factors contributing to the development of vitamin D deficiency rickets include maternal vitamin D deficiency, lack of sunlight exposure, living at high latitudes (>35° N or S of the equator), darker skin colour, wearing of head coverings and extensive skin coverage by clothing, atmospheric pollution and the non-consumption of vitamin D fortified foods. In a number of countries, such as North America, Australasia and some European countries, where vitamin D deficiency rickets has been all but eliminated, the prevalence of rickets is rising again, particularly in infants and young children of darker-skinned immigrants from Africa, the Middle East and the Indian subcontinent, and among African Americans. Recent attention has been focused on the role that vitamin D deficiency plays during pregnancy in exacerbating the risk of vitamin D deficiency rickets in breastfed infants. Although there is still no global consensus on the levels of serum 25(OH)D that reflect vitamin D sufficiency or deficiency (levels may differ depending on the function of vitamin D being studied, and on other factors such as calcium intake), low 25(OH)D concentrations are common in darker-skinned pregnant women not receiving vitamin D supplements and living in temperate climates. Cord blood 25(OH)D concentrations correlate with maternal levels but are generally lower than those in the mother, thus maternal vitamin D deficiency results in the infant being born with low 25(OH)D concentrations and an increased risk of developing hypocalcaemia and rickets unless an exogenous source of vitamin D, such as supplementation or fortified milk, is provided to the infant from birth.

Rickets due to low dietary calcium intakes may occur in the face of 25(OH)D concentrations which are generally considered to be within the normal range (>30 nmol/L), however low dietary calcium intakes may also exacerbate the development of rickets in children who have a poor vitamin D status (57). As discussed above, the pathogenesis of rickets due to low dietary calcium intakes is very similar to that of vitamin D deficiency, except that serum 1,25-dihydroxyvitamin D concentrations are typically markedly elevated in untreated patients with dietary calcium deficiency, as a consequence of the upregulation of CYP27B1 (1-alpha hydroxylase) by elevated parathyroid hormone (PTH) levels. Rickets due to low dietary calcium intakes have been described in a number of LMIC, such as South Africa, Nigeria, The Gambia, India and Bangladesh, where dairy product consumption is negligible and phytate ingestion (which binds dietary calcium) is typically high. Calcium consumption by children with active rickets in these communities has been estimated to be around 200 mg/day. Characteristically, children suffering from rickets due to low dietary calcium intakes are older than those with vitamin D deficiency. In large studies from Nigeria, the age at presentation was approximately 4 years, while in South Africa the children ranged from 4 to 16 years of age. Although low dietary calcium intakes appear to be central to the pathogenesis of nutritional rickets in these communities, it is unclear what predisposes some children to develop rickets while others with similar dietary calcium intakes do not. Genetic factors, dietary constituents besides calcium and levels of 25(OH)D may all play a role.

The study of children with active dietary calcium deficiency rickets and rachitic-like bone deformities in The Gambia has raised the possibility of another contributing factor, fibroblast growth factor 23 (FGF23) (58). Concentrations of FGF23 were markedly elevated in the children with rickets compared to community controls, and values were inversely associated with serum phosphorus and haemoglobin levels. The mechanisms by which FGF23 are elevated in the Gambian children are unclear, but it is possible that low dietary calcium intakes, through hyperparathyroidism and elevated 1,25-dihydroxyvitamin D drive the production of FGF23, which is also stimulated by chronic anaemia in the children.

Although vitamin D deficiency and dietary calcium deficiency have been discussed separately in this section, it is likely that in the majority of children with rickets the two possible aetiologies act synergistically, in that low dietary calcium intakes will aggravate the severity of rickets at a given level of 25(OH)D, while a poor vitamin D status will increase the risk of a child on a low calcium intake manifesting with bone disease. In order to eradicate the problem of nutritional rickets globally (59), a concerted effort is required to address low vitamin D status among women of childbearing age, and to ensure that at-risk infants, children and adolescents have access to vitamin D and calcium supplements, where appropriate.

CONCLUSIONS

When determining the role of diet and nutrition in healthy musculoskeletal growth and development, it is important not to assume that international recommendations are equally applicable to all populations. In addition, as new and updated evidence becomes available, it is necessary to continue to reassess those guidelines already available. It is important to gather evidence from intervention trials and from longitudinal cohorts where long-term health outcomes can be obtained. Many studies are limited by not having an 'off-treatment' follow-up period, which is an important consideration in future trial design. Reasons for lack of a response to intervention may be the timing of intervention with respect to childhood growth: some evidence suggests pre-puberty may be the opportune time for intervention, yet few trials have systematically studied children at all stages of puberty to test this hypothesis. Secondly, the populations targeted are almost always those with adequate dietary intakes of the specified nutrient, or in the case of vitamin D, adequate baseline 25(OH)D concentrations. In populations or groups of children who are particularly at risk of poor skeletal health due to nutritional deficiencies, the development of cheap, good quality and readily available diet-based and fortification strategies as well as supplement provision is paramount. Children in at-risk groups should be targeted to receive supplements, and governments should consider food fortification where appropriate, if not already in place. Importantly, existing evidence suggests that an overarching framework permitting specific advice tailored to individual populations might be the most appropriate way forward, rather than uniform global recommendations, in order to effectively reduce the global burden of musculoskeletal disease.

REFERENCES

1. WHO. *World Report on Ageing and Health 2015*. World Health Organization; 2015.
2. Aboderin IA, Beard JR. Older people's health in sub-Saharan Africa. *Lancet*. 2015;385(9968):e9-e11.
3. Oden A, McCloskey EV, Kanis JA, Harvey NC, Johansson H. Burden of high fracture probability worldwide: Secular increases 2010-2040. *Osteoporos Int*. 2015;26(9):2243-8.
4. Ward KA, Adams JE, Prentice A, Ahie-Sayer A, Cooper CC. A life course approach to healthy musculoskeletal ageing. In: Kuh D, Cooper R, Hardy R, Richards M, Ben-Shlomo Y, editors. *A Life Course Approach to Ageing*. Oxford: Oxford University Press; 2014:162-77.
5. Heaney R, Abrams S, Dawson-Highes B, Looker A, Marcus R, Matkovic V, et al. Peak bone mass. *Osteoporos Int*. 2000;11(12):985-1009.

6. Cooper C, Campion G, Melton LJ, 3rd. Hip fractures in the elderly: A world-wide projection. *Osteoporos Int.* 1992;2(6):285-9.

7. Carter D, Bouxsein M, Marcus R. New approaches for interpreting projected bone densitometry data. *J Bone Miner Res.* 1992;7:137-45.

8. Crabtree NJ, Kibirige MS, Fordham JN, Banks LM, Muntoni F, Chinn D, et al. The relationship between lean body mass and bone mineral content in paediatric health and disease. *Bone.* 2004;35(4):965-72.

9. Hogler W, Briody J, Woodhead HJ, Chan A, Cowell CT. Importance of lean mass in the interpretation of total body densitometry in children and adolescents. *J Pediatr.* 2003;143(1):81-8.

10. Kroger H, Vainio P, Nieminen J, Kotaniemi A. Comparison of different models for interpreting bone mineral density measurements using DXA and MRI technology. *Bone.* 1995;17(2):157-9.

11. Prentice A, Parsons T, Cole T. Uncritical use of bone mineral density in absorptiometry may lead to size-related artifacts in the identification of bone mineral determinants. *Am J Clin Nutr.* 1994;60:837-42.

12. Zemel BS, Leonard MB, Kelly A, Lappe JM, Gilsanz V, Oberfield S, et al. Height adjustment in assessing dual energy x-ray absorptiometry measurements of bone mass and density in children. *J Clin Endocrinol Metab.* 2010;95(3):1265-73.

13. Molgaard C, Thomsen B, Prentice A, Cole T, Michealsen K. Whole body bone mineral content in healthy children and adolescents. *Arch Dis Child.* 1997;76:9-15.

14. Zemel BS, Kalkwarf HJ, Gilsanz V, Lappe JM, Oberfield S, Shepherd JA, et al. Revised reference curves for bone mineral content and areal bone mineral density according to age and sex for black and non-black children: Results of the bone mineral density in childhood study. *J Clin Endocrinol Metab.* 2011;96(10):3160-9.

15. Bishop N, Arundel P, Clark E, Dimitri P, Farr J, Jones G, et al. Fracture prediction and the definition of osteoporosis in children and adolescents: The ISCD 2013 Pediatric Official Positions. *J Clin Densitom.* 2014;17(2):275-80.

16. Crabtree NJ, Arabi A, Bachrach LK, Fewtrell M, El-Hajj Fuleihan G, Kecskemethy HH, et al. Dual-energy X-ray absorptiometry interpretation and reporting in children and adolescents: The revised 2013 ISCD Pediatric Official Positions. *J Clin Densitom.* 2014;17(2):225-42.

17. Adams JE, Engelke K, Zemel BS, Ward KA. Quantitative computer tomography in children and adolescents: The 2013 ISCD Pediatric Official Positions. *J Clin Densitom.* 2014;17(2):258-74.

18. Ward K. Musculoskeletal phenotype through the life course: The role of nutrition. *Proc Nutr Soc.* 2012;71(1):27-37.

19. Bailey D, McKay H, Mirwald R, Crocker P, Faulkner R. A six-year longitudinal study of the relationship of physical activity to bone mineral accrual in growing children: The University of Saskatchewan bone mineral accrual study. *J Bone Miner Res.* 1999;14(10):1672-9.

20. Baxter-Jones ADG, Faulkner RA, Forwood MR, Mirwald RL, Bailey DA. Bone mineral accrual from 8 to 30 years of age: An estimation of peak bone mass. *J Bone Miner Res.* 2011;26(8):1729-39.

21. Cooper C, Eriksson JG, Forsen T, Osmond C, Tuomilehto J, Barker DJ. Maternal height, childhood growth and risk of hip fracture in later life: A longitudinal study. *Osteoporos Int.* 2001;12(8):623-9.

22. Javaid MK, Lekamwasam S, Clark J, Dennison EM, Syddall HE, Loveridge N, et al. Infant growth influences proximal femoral geometry in adulthood. *J Bone Miner Res.* 2006;21(4):508-12.

23. Javaid MK, Eriksson JG, Kajantie E, Forsen T, Osmond C, Barker DJ, et al. Growth in childhood predicts hip fracture risk in later life. *Osteoporos Int.* 2011;22(1):69-73.

24. Cole TJ, Kuh D, Johnson W, Ward KA, Howe LD, Adams JE, et al. Using Super-Imposition by Translation And Rotation (SITAR) to relate pubertal growth to bone health in later life: The Medical Research Council (MRC) National Survey of Health and Development. *Int J Epidemiol.* 2016;45(4):1125-34.

25. Kuh D, Muthuri SG, Moore A, Cole TJ, Adams JE, Cooper C, et al. Pubertal timing and bone phenotype in early old age: Findings from a British birth cohort study. *Int J Epidemiol.* 2016;45(4):1113-24.

26. Kuh D, Wills AK, Shah I, Prentice A, Hardy R, Adams JE, et al. Growth from birth to adulthood and bone phenotype in early old age: A British birth cohort study. *J Bone Miner Res.* 2014;29(1):123-33.

27. Kuh D, Pierce M, Adams J, Deanfield J, Ekelund U, Friberg P, et al. Cohort profile: Updating the cohort profile for the MRC National Survey of Health and Development: A new clinic-based data collection for ageing research. *Int J Epidemiol.* 2011;40(1):e1-9.

28. Tandon N, Fall CH, Osmond C, Sachdev HP, Prabhakaran D, Ramakrishnan L, et al. Growth from birth to adulthood and peak bone mass and density data from the New Delhi Birth Cohort. *Osteoporos Int.* 2012;23(10):2447-59.

29. Prentice A. Diet, nutrition and the prevention of osteoporosis. *Public Health Nutr.* 2004;7(1A):227-43.

30. Lappe JM, Watson P, Gilsanz V, Hangartner T, Kalkwarf HJ, Oberfield S, et al. The longitudinal effects of physical activity and dietary calcium on bone mass accrual across stages of pubertal development. *J Bone Miner Res.* 2015;30(1):156-64.

31. Matsuzaki M, Kuper H, Kulkarni B, Radhakrishna KV, Viljakainen H, Taylor AE, et al. Life-course determinants of bone mass in young adults from a transitional rural community in India: The Andhra Pradesh Children and Parents Study (APCAPS). *Am J Clin Nutr.* 2014;99(6):1450-9.

32. Bonjour J, Carrie A, Ferrari S, Clavien H, Slosman D, Theintz G, et al. Calcium-enriched foods and bone mass growth in prepubertal girls: A randomized, double blind, placebo-controlled trial. *J Clin Invest.* 1997;99(6):1287-94.

33. Bonjour JP, Chevally T, Ammann P, Slosman D, Rizzoli R. Gain in bone mass in prepubertal girls 3.5 years after discontinuation of calcium supplementation: A follow-up study. *Lancet.* 2001;358:1208-12.

34. Cadogan J, Eastell R, Jones N, Barker ME. Milk intake and bone mineral acquisition in adolescent girls: Randomised, controlled intervention trial. *BMJ (Clin Res Ed).* 1997;315(7118):1255-60.

35. Dibba B, Prentice A, Ceesay M, Mendy M, Darboe S, Stirling DM, et al. Bone mineral contents and plasma osteocalcin concentrations of Gambian children 12 and 24 mo after the withdrawal of a calcium supplement. *Am J Clin Nutr.* 2002;76(3):681-6.

36. Dibba B, Prentice A, Ceesay M, Stirling DM, Cole TJ, Poskitt EM. Effect of calcium supplementation on bone mineral accretion in Gambian children accustomed to a low-calcium diet. *Am J Clin Nutr.* 2000;71(2):544-9.

37. Lambert HL, Eastell R, Karnik K, Russell JM, Barker ME. Calcium supplementation and bone mineral accretion in adolescent girls: An 18-mo randomized controlled trial with 2-y follow-up. *Am J Clin Nutr.* 2008;87(2):455-62.

38. Specker BL. Evidence for an interaction between caclium intake and physical activity on changes in bone mineral density. *J Bone Miner Res.* 1996;11(10):1539-44.

39. Ward KA, Roberts SA, Adams JE, Lanham-New S, Mughal MZ. Calcium supplementation and weight bearing physical activity – Do they have a combined effect on the bone density of pre-pubertal children? *Bone.* 2007;41(4):496-504.

40. Winzenberg T, Shaw K, Fryer J, Jones G. Effects of calcium supplementation on bone density in healthy children: Meta-analysis of randomised controlled trials. *BMJ (Clin Res Ed).* 2006;333(7572):775.

41. Chevalley T, Rizzoli R, Hans D, Ferrari S, Bonjour JP. Interaction between calcium intake and menarcheal age on bone mass gain: An eight-year follow-up study from prepuberty to postmenarche. *J Clin Endocrinol Metab.* 2005;90(1):44-51.

42. Prentice A, Dibba B, Sawo Y, Cole TJ. The effect of prepubertal calcium carbonate supplementation on the age of peak height velocity in Gambian adolescents. *Am J Clin Nutr.* 2012;96(5):1042-50.

43. Ward KA, Cole TJ, Laskey MA, Ceesay M, Mendy MB, Sawo Y, et al. The effect of prepubertal calcium carbonate supplementation on skeletal development in Gambian boys-a 12-year follow-up study. *J Clin Endocrinol Metab.* 2014;99(9):3169-76.

44. Budek AZ, Hoppe C, Ingstrup H, Michaelsen KF, Bugel S, Molgaard C. Dietary protein intake and bone mineral content in adolescents – The Copenhagen Cohort Study. *Osteoporos Int.* 2007;18(12):1661-7.

45. Zhu K, Du X, Cowell CT, Greenfield H, Blades B, Dobbins TA, et al. Effects of school milk intervention on cortical bone accretion and indicators relevant to bone metabolism in Chinese girls aged 10-12 y in Beijing. *Am J Clin Nutr.* 2005;81(5):1168-75.

46. Zhu K, Zhang Q, Foo LH, Trube A, Ma G, Hu X, et al. Growth, bone mass, and vitamin D status of Chinese adolescent girls 3 y after withdrawal of milk supplementation. *Am J Clin Nutr.* 2006;83(3):714-21.

47. Umaretiya PJ, Thacher TD, Fischer PR, Cha SS, Pettifor JM. Bone mineral density in Nigerian children after discontinuation of calcium supplementation. *Bone.* 2013;55(1):64-8.

48. Ward KA, Cole TJ, Laskey MA, Ceesay M, Mendy MB, Prentice A. The effect of calcium supplementation on adolescent bone growth in pre-pubertal Gambian females: A 12-year follow-up study. *Bone Abstracts.* 2015(4):42.

49. Institute of Medicine. *Dietary Reference Intakes for Calcium and Vitamin D.* Ross AC, Taylor CL, Yaktine AL, Del Valle HB, editors. Washington DC: Institute of Medicine; 2010.

50. Scientific Advisory Committee on Nutrition. *Vitamin D and Health Report.* London: Public Health England; July 2016.

51. Winzenberg T, Powell S, Shaw KA, Jones G. Effects of vitamin D supplementation on bone density in healthy children: Systematic review and meta-analysis. *BMJ (Clin Res Ed).* 2011;342:c7254.

52. El-Hajj Fuleihan G, Nabulsi M, Tamim H, Maalouf J, Salamoun M, Khalife H, et al. Effect of vitamin D replacement on musculoskeletal parameters in school children: A randomized controlled trial. *J Clin Endocrinol Metab.* 2006;91(2):405-12.

53. Ghazal N, Al-Shaar L, Maalouf J, Nabulsi M, Arabi A, Choucair M, et al. Persistent effect of vitamin D supplementation on musculoskeletal parameters in adolescents one year after trial completion. *J Bone Miner Res.* 2016;31(7):1473-80.

54. Ward KA, Das G, Roberts SA, Berry JL, Adams JE, Rawer R, et al. A randomized, controlled trial of vitamin D supplementation upon musculoskeletal health in postmenarchal females. *J Clin Endocrinol Metab.* 2010;95(10):4643-51.

55. Khadilkar AV, Sayyad MG, Sanwalka NJ, Bhandari DR, Naik S, Khadilkar VV, et al. Vitamin D supplementation and bone mass accrual in under-privileged adolescent Indian girls. *Asia Pac J Clin Nutr.* 2010;19(4):465-72.

56. Sanwalka N, Khadilkar A, Chiplonkar S, Khatod K, Phadke N, Khadilkar V. Influence of vitamin D receptor gene Fok1 polymorphism on bone mass accrual post calcium and vitamin D supplementation. *Indian J Pediatr.* 2015;82(11):985-90.

57. Pettifor JM. Calcium and vitamin D metabolism in children in developing countries. *Ann Nutr Metab.* 2014;64(Suppl. 2):15-22.

58. Prentice A. Nutritional rickets around the world. *J Steroid Biochem Mol Biol.* 2013;136:201-6

59. Munns CF, Shaw N, Kiely M, Specker BL, Thacher TD, Ozono K, et al. Global consensus recommendations on prevention and management of nutritional rickets. *J Clin Endocrinol Metab.* 2016;101(2):394-415.

7

Developmental plasticity, epigenetic mechanisms and early life influences on adult health and disease: Fundamental concepts

ELIZABETH M CURTIS, KAREN LILLYCROP
AND MARK HANSON

INTRODUCTION

Osteoporosis, which is characterised by low bone mass, poor bone structure and an increased risk of fracture, has been suggested to result in part from impaired osteoblast cell proliferation, differentiation or function in early development. Bone formation is dependent upon mesenchymal stem cells (MSCs) which can differentiate to form osteoblasts. Bone development and remodelling is then maintained through a balance between the bone-forming osteoblasts and the bone-resorbing osteoclasts.

Although studies of twins and family linkage studies have shown some fixed genetic variants which contribute to the inheritance of bone mineral density and fracture risk, the heritability (i.e. the extent to which the variation in phenotype in the population can be explained by fixed genetic differences) is not high and the variance in BMD between individuals is only partly explained by these genetic factors (1–3). There is increasing evidence that much of the variance in both BMD and fracture risk might be explained by the influence of the environment on gene expression, both in utero and in early life (4). It is widely recognised that genes effectively provide a library of information that can be read (expressed) differently in different cells and at different times according to function and need. Thus in a single organism, although the genetic code contained in every somatic cell is the same, the genes expressed will vary widely from organ to organ and even from cell to cell, often in response to environmental cues (5). This regulation of gene expression is now recognised to involve a range of epigenetic processes.

INTRODUCTION TO EPIGENETIC MECHANISMS

The processes of developmental plasticity – by which a single genotype may give rise to several different phenotypes in response to the prevailing environmental milieu – is ubiquitous in the natural world. This process allows the next generation to be born appropriately adapted to the expected external environment, using cues from the prevailing environmental conditions acting during critical periods of development (6). A widely reported example is the meadow vole (*Microtus pennsylvanicus*), in which the thickness of the coat in the offspring is determined by the photoperiod (number of hours of light and dark) experienced by the mother during gestation. Pups born in autumn have a thicker coat than those born in spring (7). Maternal melatonin levels during pregnancy are the most likely signal to the pup the prevailing environmental conditions (8), allowing the pup to adopt a developmental trajectory appropriate to the postnatal environment to which it is likely to be exposed after birth. However, a mismatch between the expected postnatal environment and that to which the pup has been developmentally programmed, for example due to a change in the postnatal environment or inappropriate maternal cues, would lead to a survival disadvantage (9).

A range of experimental studies have shown that alterations to maternal diet during pregnancy may lead to changes in offspring phenotype and gene expression (10,11). These effects are likely to be underpinned by epigenetic mechanisms, processes by which gene expression is modified but without changes in the DNA code itself. Such epigenetic signals are essential in determining when and where genes are expressed. They can be conserved across multiple generations, as has been shown following exposure to environmental chemicals, but also can be reinstated de novo in each generation (12,13). In humans, most epigenetic effects have only been shown to pass to the grandchildren, which does not prove a transgenerational effect, as epigenetic effects can be induced in the primordial germ cells of the F1 during F0 pregnancy and produce effects in the F2 generation (14,15). The epigenome can, however, be regarded as a molecular record of life events, accumulating throughout a lifetime. For example, monozygotic twins have been shown to be epigenetically most similar at birth but their epigenomes diverge with age at a rate that is lessened if they share a common environment (16). An understanding of these epigenetic processes has the potential to enable early intervention strategies to improve early development and later health; consequently, the study of epigenetic biomarkers is a rapidly advancing field (17).

Epigenetic mechanisms include DNA methylation, histone modifications and non-coding RNAs (ncRNAs), as shown in Figure 7.1 (5,18–20).

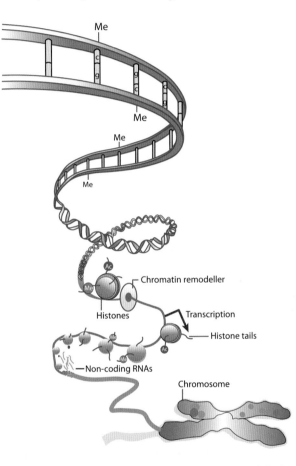

Figure 7.1 The coding and structural information superimposed the base sequence of DNA is organised in multiple epigenomes, which differ according to cell and tissue type. DNA methylation at cytosine adjacent to guanine bases (CpG sites), in addition to the covalent modifications of histone tails and histone variants, can contribute information to nucleosomal remodelling machines. (Nucleosomes are a subunit of DNA packaging composed of eight histone protein cores forming a complex around which DNA is wrapped.) Through nucleosome remodelling, leading to ravelling and unravelling of DNA, genes and loci encoding non-coding RNAs become susceptible to transcription. Transcription factors (not shown in this diagram) also play a major part in the competence and organisation of the genome. (Reproduced from Jones PA et al., *Nature*. 2008;454(7205):711-5.)

POST-TRANSLATIONAL HISTONE MODIFICATIONS

Post-translational histone modifications and the accompanying histone-modifying enzymes form a major part of the epigenetic regulation of genes. DNA is wrapped around an octamer of four different histone molecules (H2A, H2B, H3 and H4) to form a nucleosome, the basic unit of chromatin. The flexible N-terminal tails of core histones that protrude from the nucleosome undergo various post-translational modifications, including acetylation, methylation, phosphorylation, ubiquitination, sumoylation, ADP ribosylation, deamination and noncovalent proline isomerization (21). The patterns of histone modifications alter the transcriptional accessibility of the chromatin. It has been shown that euchromatin, a more relaxed, actively transcribed state of DNA, is characterized by high levels of acetylation and trimethylated (H3) lysine residues (K-number) on specific histones H3K4, H3K36 and H3K79, while low levels of acetylation and high levels of H3K9, H3K27 and H4K20 methylation are indicative of a more condensed, transcriptionally inactive heterochromatin (22). The majority of histone post-translational modifications are dynamic and regulated by families of enzymes that promote or reverse specific modifications, such as histone acetyltransferases (HATs), which add acetylation marks, whereas histone deacetylases (HDACs) remove them. Many transcriptional co-activators or co-repressors possess either HAT or HDAC activity or associate with these enzymes, so the balance between histone methylation and acetylation and demethylation/deacetylation is important in modifying expression of target genes.

NON-CODING RNAs

Recent studies have shown that up to 90% of the eukaryotic genome is transcribed, but only 1% to 2% of the genome encodes proteins (1,23). In recent years, it has become increasingly apparent that the nonprotein-coding portion of the genome plays a crucial role in the control of biological processes such as proliferation, differentiation and apoptosis. Micro RNAs (miRNAs) are the best characterised ncRNAs, approximately 21 nucleotide-long noncoding RNA molecules. miRNAs are incorporated into an RNA-induced silencing complex (RISC) in order to facilitate binding to the target mRNA, usually within its 3′ untranslated region. If the miRNA and the target RNA match, this results in the degradation of the targeted transcript. More commonly, miRNAs bind imperfectly to their targets, causing translational repression only, without the destruction of mRNA. In general, miRNAs are considered predominantly as negative regulators of gene expression involved in physiological and pathological processes; however, some have been shown to activate translation under certain conditions (24,25).

miRNAs are, however, part of a larger family of ncRNAs, which includes small nucleolar RNAs and long ncRNAs (lncRNAs). The lncRNAs make up the largest portion of the mammalian noncoding transcriptome, but their mechanism of action is still not fully understood. Studies have shown they can regulate gene expression by acting as either antisense transcripts or as scaffolds for the recruitment of histone modifiers (7,26).

DNA METHYLATION

DNA methylation is the most widely studied of epigenetic modifications and is the focus of this chapter – although there is experimental evidence for the role of miRNAs and histone modifications in the regulation of bone development, and it is likely that all three epigenetic processes work in concert to control gene expression. DNA methylation is a common modification in eukaryotic organisms, and involves the transfer of a methyl group to the 5′ carbon position of cytosine, creating 5-methylcytosine (5-mC) (27). It is a relatively stable epigenetic mark that can be transmitted through DNA replication during mitosis (28), although methyl marks can be added and removed throughout the lifecourse. Cytosine methylation mainly occurs within the dinucleotide sequence CpG, where a cytosine is immediately 5′ to a guanine, with a phosphate group between them denoted by 'p', although non-CpG methylation is also prevalent in embryonic stem cells (29). A CpG site can be either methylated or unmethylated in an individual cell; however, across a whole tissue where a particular site may be methylated or unmethylated in a large number of cells, a range of graded gene expression from 0% to 100% is possible (5).

CpG dinucleotides are not randomly distributed throughout the genome but are clustered at the 5′ end of genes in regions known as CpG islands, with hypermethylation of CpG islands generally associated with gene silencing and hypomethylation with activation (30). DNA methylation can act directly to block binding of transcription factors to the DNA or by recruiting a myriad of other repressive factors, such as methyl CpG–binding protein 2 (MeCP2), which in turn mediate local chromatin changes to impair transcription factor binding (31). The pattern of CpG methylation is largely established during embryogenesis, fetal and perinatal life. DNA methylation marks on the maternal and paternal genomes are largely erased on fertilisation (with the exception of the imprinted genes and other specific genomic regions), followed by a wave of *de novo* methylation within the inner cell mass just prior to blastocyst implantation (32,33). The *de novo* methylation of DNA is catalysed by DNA methyltransferases (DNMT) 3a and 3b (33), and is maintained through mitosis by methylation of hemi-methylated DNA by DNA methyltransferase 1 (DNMT1) (34). This enables lineage-specific methylation patterns to be maintained in differentiated tissues. DNA methylation was initially thought to be relatively stable and generally maintained throughout life, but this concept has now been challenged. In 2009 the existence of another epigenetic modification, 5-hydroxymethylcytosine (5hmC), was described as present in high levels in neurons and embryonic stem (ES) cells (35). 5hmC has been shown to arise from the oxidation of 5-mC by the enzymes of the ten-eleven-translocation (TET) family (36) and has been proposed to act as a specific epigenetic mark opposing DNA methylation, as well as a passive intermediate in the demethylation pathway (37,38). The high levels found in the brain and neurons indicate a role in the control of neuronal differentiation and neuronal plasticity (39).

EARLY LIFE NUTRITION AND MODIFICATIONS TO THE EPIGENOME

Although DNA methylation was originally thought to be a very stable modification, and once established, methylation patterns were largely maintained throughout the lifecourse, there is now growing evidence that a number of environmental factors such as nutrition, stress, placental insufficiency, endocrine disruptors and pollution, especially in early life, can alter the epigenome, leading to long-term phenotypic changes in the offspring (40).

One of the best examples of how nutrition can alter phenotype through the altered epigenetic regulation of genes is seen in studies on the honeybee. Female larvae incubated in the presence of royal jelly predominantly develop into queen bees, while those incubated in the absence of royal jelly develop into sterile worker bees, even though they are genetically identical (41,42). However, knockdown of DNA methyltransferase 3 (DNMT3), the major DNA methyl transferase in bees, increased the proportion of larvae developing into queen bees as opposed to sterile workers (42). Nutrition has also been shown to influence DNA methylation in rodents. In A^{vy} mice, coat colour is determined by the methylation status of an intracisternal-A particle (IAP) in the 5′ upstream region of the agouti gene. Supplementation of the maternal diet with folic acid, cobalamin, choline and betaine induced a graded shift in coat colour of the litter from predominately yellow (agouti) to brown (pseudo-agouti) (43). This shift was accompanied by the hypermethylation of seven CpG dinucleotides 600 bp downstream of the A^{vy} IAP insertion site. There is also evidence from models of nutritional programming that early life nutrition can induce persistent epigenetic and phenotypic changes in the offspring. For example, feeding pregnant rats a protein restricted (PR) diet induced hypomethylation of the glucocorticoid receptor (GR) and peroxisome proliferator–activated receptor (PPAR)α promoters in the livers of juvenile and adult offspring; this was accompanied by an increase in GR and PPARα expression and in the metabolic processes that they control (44–46). In contrast, global dietary restriction during pregnancy increased the level of DNA methylation of PPARα and the GR in the liver of the offspring (47), suggesting that the effects of maternal nutrition on the epigenome of the offspring depend upon the nature of the maternal nutrient challenge. Such nutrition-related responses are consistent with the concept that induced epigenetic changes that underpin physiological change may provide a means of adapting to an adverse environment (48). Such effects are not limited to nutrient restriction, as high fat diets have also been shown to induce methylation changes in the offspring. Vucetic et al. showed increased expression of the μ-opioid receptor (MOR) and preproenkephalin (PENK) in the nucleus accumbens, prefrontal cortex and hypothalamus of mice from dams that consumed the high fat (HF) diet during pregnancy, and this was accompanied by the hypomethylation of the promoter regions of these genes (49).

Studies in animal models, where the diet pre- and post-pregnancy as well as genetic background can be carefully controlled, have been instrumental in demonstrating long-term effects of nutrition on the epigeneome. Evidence that maternal diet in humans can induce long-term epigenetic and phenotypic changes in the offspring is more limited. However, in humans, alterations have been reported in the methylation of a number of genes in DNA isolated from whole blood from individuals whose mothers were exposed to famine during the Dutch Hunger Winter. The timing of the nutritional constraint appeared to be important, as exposure to famine around the time of conception was associated with a small decrease in CpG methylation of the imprinted *IGF2* gene and an increase in methylation of leptin, *IL-10*, *MEG3* and *ABCA4* (50), while late gestation famine exposure had no effect on methylation. This study also provided evidence that maternal nutritional constraint induces long-term epigenetic changes in key metabolic regulatory genes, as these measurements were made 60 years after the famine exposure. Studies of dietary supplementation with 400µg of folic acid per day around the time of conception have also shown altered methylation of specific CpG sites in the *IGF2* gene in the peripheral blood cells of children (51). There is also some evidence that plasticity in the human epigenome may persist into adulthood, as, for example, short-term high fat overfeeding in healthy young men was shown to induce methylation changes in over 6000 skeletal muscle genes, with only partial reversal after 6 to 8 weeks of a normocaloric diet (52).

EFFECTS OF ENVIRONMENTAL INSULTS AND AGEING ON DNA METHYLATION

Smoking is a well-recognised exposure which is associated with methylation modifications in DNA, demonstrated in many epigenome-wide association studies (EWAS), summarised in a subsequent meta-analysis (53). Indeed, DNA methylation patterns can be used as biomarkers of smoking exposure for research and clinical practice.

Age-related changes in DNA methylation are well documented. Various studies have worked towards an understanding of epigenetic predictors of ageing and mortality, using methylation measures from multiple CpG sites across the genome to predict chronological age in humans (54,55). Hannum *et al.* created an age predictor based on a single cohort in which DNA methylation was measured in whole blood (54), while Horvath developed an age predictor using DNA methylation data from multiple studies (including the Hannum dataset) and multiple tissues (55). In both studies, the difference between methylation-predicted age and chronological age (that is, Δ_{age}) was proposed as an index of disproportionate 'biological' aging and was hypothesised to be associated with risk for age-related diseases and mortality. Other studies have shown that this Δ_{age}, or marker of accelerated ageing, can be used to predict mortality independently of health status, lifestyle factors and known genetic factors (56,57).

EPIGENETIC MARKS AS BIOMARKERS

The association between early life exposures and epigenetic changes in key metabolic regulatory genes suggests that such changes may well underpin the long-term changes in gene expression and metabolism seen in the offspring. However, because of the technical challenges associated with changing the methylation status of a single CpG site in vivo, there is as yet no formal proof that these methylation changes are causal. Although whether causally involved in the development of a disease or a bystander effect of a change in phenotype, the detection of such methylation changes may provide useful markers to identify individuals at increased risk of disease. Consistent with this paradigm, Godfrey et al. reported in two independent cohorts that the methylation status of a single CpG site in the promoter region of the retinoid X receptor A (RXRA) was related positively to childhood adiposity in both boys and girls such that RXRA promoter methylation explained over a fifth of the variance in childhood fat mass (58), while Clarke-Harris et al. demonstrated that the methylation of CpG sites in the promoter of PGC1a in peripheral blood at age 5 to 7 years were predictive of adiposity in the children at ages 9 to 14 (59).

These findings not only support the hypothesis that developmentally induced epigenetic marks make a significant contribution to later phenotype but also suggest that the detection of epigenetic marks even in peripheral tissue may allow identification of individuals at increased risk of chronic disease in later life before the onset of clinical disease.

However, a number of challenges remain. First, tissue samples commonly used in EWAS studies such as blood, fat, placenta and umbilical cord tissue are made up of multiple cell types, and a change in methylation may represent a change in the proportion of cell types within the tissues rather than an intrinsic change in methylation within the cells. Algorithms have been developed to account for such differences, although whether the methylation signal determined by cell mix should be discarded is questionable, as such a change in cell type may be extremely relevant to the disease phenotype. Secondly, DNA methylation has been assessed using a variety of methods, making comparison between studies difficult and the identification of robust markers of phenotype limited. The cost of the genome-wide methylation approaches has also been high, resulting often in small numbers of subjects being studied. However, with the development of Illumina Human Methylation 450K BeadChip, and more recently the EPIC array, which provide a relatively cost-effective method to look for 'genome-wide' methylation differences, many researchers are increasingly using these platforms to measure DNA methylation, which will allow comparisons between studies and the potential to combine data across many thousands of data sets. However, it should be noted that even with EPIC arrays only a very small percentage of the CpGs within the genome are covered.

Notwithstanding these caveats, detection of DNA methylation changes in early life provides an opportunity to identify individuals at increased risk of disease and, as DNA methylation reflects both genotype and environment, a more powerful biomarker than genotype or environment alone. Such epigenetic biomarkers may also provide immediate outcome measures to evaluate potential prenatal interventions as well as provide new insights into postnatal exposures that can change these epigenetic marks and perhaps disease risk. Thus, it may be possible to not only identify those at risk of developing later disease through the use of epigenetic biomarkers early in life, but to develop intervention strategies which target and reverse these epigenetic changes.

CONCLUSIONS

There is now considerable evidence that our genotype and later environment are not the only determinants of noncommunicable disease (NCD) risk, and that epigenetic marks induced by the early life environment are associated with altered gene expression patterns in important metabolic tissues, leading to altered susceptibility to disease in later life.

Demonstration of a role for altered epigenetic regulation of genes in the development of NCDs together with the identification of potential epigenetic biomarkers of future disease risk raises the possibility of preventive medicine. Individuals identified as at-risk at an early stage in the lifecourse could receive nutritional or lifestyle interventions, allowing a more effective strategy of preventive treatment. This would both improve quality of life and reduce the economic burden associated with current treatment strategies. Further understanding of the mechanisms by which nutrition can modify the epigenome and the periods of epigenetic susceptibility may aid development of novel intervention strategies to reverse this current global epidemic of NCDs such as osteoporosis.

REFERENCES

1. Richards JB, Zheng HF, Spector TD. Genetics of osteoporosis from genome-wide association studies: Advances and challenges. *Nat Rev Genet.* 2012;13(8):576-88.
2. Zheng HF, Forgetta V, Hsu YH, Estrada K, Rosello-Diez A, Leo PJ, et al. Whole-genome sequencing identifies EN1 as a determinant of bone density and fracture. *Nature.* 2015;526(7571):112-7.
3. Yang J, Bakshi A, Zhu Z, Hemani G, Vinkhuyzen AA, Lee SH, et al. Genetic variance estimation with imputed variants finds negligible missing heritability for human height and body mass index. *Nat Genet.* 2015;47(10):1114-20.
4. Dennison EM, Arden NK, Keen RW, Syddall H, Day IN, Spector TD, et al. Birthweight, vitamin D receptor genotype and the programming of osteoporosis. *Paediatr Perinat Epidemiol.* 2001;15(3):211-9.
5. Gluckman PD, Hanson MA, Cooper C, Thornburg KL. Effect of in utero and early-life conditions on adult health and disease. *N Engl J Med.* 2008;359(1):61-73.
6. Hanson MA, Gluckman PD. Early Developmental conditioning of later health and disease: Physiology or pathophysiology? *Physiol Rev.* 2014;94(4):1027-76.

7. Lee TM, Zucker I. Vole infant development is influenced perinatally by maternal photoperiodic history. *Am J Physiol.* 1988;255(5 Pt 2):R831-8.

8. Lee TM, Spears N, Tuthill CR, Zucker I. Maternal melatonin treatment influences rates of neonatal development of meadow vole pups. *Biol Reprod.* 1989;40(3):495-502.

9. Godfrey KM, Lillycrop KA, Burdge GC, Gluckman PD, Hanson MA. Epigenetic mechanisms and the mismatch concept of the developmental origins of health and disease. *Pediatr Res.* 2007;61(5 Pt 2):5R-10R.

10. Lillycrop KA, Phillips ES, Jackson AA, Hanson MA, Burdge GC. Dietary protein restriction of pregnant rats induces and folic acid supplementation prevents epigenetic modification of hepatic gene expression in the offspring. *J Nutr.* 2005;135(6):1382-6.

11. Burdge GC, Slater-Jefferies J, Torrens C, Phillips ES, Hanson MA, Lillycrop KA. Dietary protein restriction of pregnant rats in the F0 generation induces altered methylation of hepatic gene promoters in the adult male offspring in the F1 and F2 generations. *Br J Nutr.* 2007;97(3):435-9.

12. Hanson MA, Skinner MK. Developmental origins of epigenetic transgenerational inheritance. *Environ Epigenet.* 2016;2(1):dvw002.

13. Burdge GC, Hoile SP, Uller T, Thomas NA, Gluckman PD, Hanson MA, et al. Progressive, transgenerational changes in offspring phenotype and epigenotype following nutritional transition. *PloS One.* 2011; 6(11):e28282.

14. Jaenisch R, Bird A. Epigenetic regulation of gene expression: How the genome integrates intrinsic and environmental signals. *Nat Genet.* 2003;33 Suppl:245-54.

15. Grossniklaus U, Kelly WG, Ferguson-Smith AC, Pembrey M, Lindquist S. Transgenerational epigenetic inheritance: How important is it? *Nat Rev Genet.* 2013;14(3):228-35.

16. Fraga MF, Ballestar E, Paz MF, Ropero S, Setien F, Ballestar ML, et al. Epigenetic differences arise during the lifetime of monozygotic twins. *Proc Natl Acad Sci U S A.* 2005;102(30):10604-9.

17. Godfrey KM, Costello PM, Lillycrop KA. The developmental environment, epigenetic biomarkers and long-term health. *J Dev Orig Health Dis.* 2015;6(5):399-406.

18. Gicquel C, El-Osta A, Le Bouc Y. Epigenetic regulation and fetal programming. *Best Pract Res Clin Endocrinol Metab.* 2008;22(1):1-16.

19. Tang WY, Ho SM. Epigenetic reprogramming and imprinting in origins of disease. *Rev Endocr Metab Disord.* 2007;8(2):173-82.

20. American Association for Cancer Research Human Epinome Task Force, et al. Moving AHEAD with an international human epigenome project. *Nature.* 2008;454(7205):711-5.

21. Gibney ER, Nolan CM. Epigenetics and gene expression. *Heredity.* 2010;105(1):4-13.

22. Portela A, Esteller M. Epigenetic modifications and human disease. *Nature Biotechnol.* 2010;28(10):1057-68.

23. Consortium EP, Birney E, Stamatoyannopoulos JA, Dutta A, Guigo R, Gingeras TR, et al. Identification and analysis of functional elements in 1% of the human genome by the ENCODE pilot project. *Nature.* 2007;447(7146):799-816.

24. Huntzinger E, Izaurralde E. Gene silencing by microRNAs: Contributions of translational repression and mRNA decay. *Nat Rev Genet.* 2011;12(2):99-110.

25. Kapinas K, Delany AM. MicroRNA biogenesis and regulation of bone remodeling. *Arthritis Res Ther.* 2011;13(3):220.

26. Esteller M. Non-coding RNAs in human disease. *Nat Rev Genet.* 2011;12(12):861-74.

27. Kumar S, Cheng X, Klimasauskas S, Mi S, Posfai J, Roberts RJ, et al. The DNA (cytosine-5) methyltransferases. *Nucleic Acids Res.* 1994;22(1):1-10.

28. Bird A. DNA methylation patterns and epigenetic memory. *Genes Dev.* 2002;16(1):6-21.

29. Ramsahoye BH, Biniszkiewicz D, Lyko F, Clark V, Bird AP, Jaenisch R. Non-CpG methylation is prevalent in embryonic stem cells and may be mediated by DNA methyltransferase 3a. *Proc Natl Acad Sci U S A.* 2000;97(10):5237-42.

30. Song F, Smith JF, Kimura MT, Morrow AD, Matsuyama T, Nagase H, et al. Association of tissue-specific differentially methylated regions (TDMs) with differential gene expression. *Proc Natl Acad Sci U S A.* 2005;102(9):3336-41.

31. Fuks F, Hurd PJ, Wolf D, Nan X, Bird AP, Kouzarides T. The methyl-CpG-binding protein MeCP2 links DNA methylation to histone methylation. *J Biol Chem.* 2003;278(6):4035-40.

32. Okano M, Bell DW, Haber DA, Li E. DNA methyltransferases Dnmt3a and Dnmt3b are essential for de novo methylation and mammalian development. *Cell.* 1999;99(3):247-57.

33. Santos F, Hendrich B, Reik W, Dean W. Dynamic reprogramming of DNA methylation in the early mouse embryo. *Dev Biol.* JID-0372762. 2002;241(1):172-82.

34. Bacolla A, Pradhan S, Roberts RJ, Wells RD. Recombinant human DNA (cytosine-5) methyltransferase. II. Steady-state kinetics reveal allosteric activation by methylated dna. *J Biol Chem.* 1999;274(46):33011-9.

35. Tahiliani M, Koh KP, Shen Y, Pastor WA, Bandukwala H, Brudno Y, et al. Conversion of 5-methylcytosine to 5-hydroxymethylcytosine in mammalian DNA by MLL partner TET1. *Science.* 2009;324(5929):930-5.

36. Ito S, Shen L, Dai Q, Wu SC, Collins LB, Swenberg JA, et al. TET proteins can convert 5-methylcytosine to 5-formylcytosine and 5-carboxylcytosine. *Science.* 2011;333(6047):1300-3.

37. Guibert S, Weber M. Functions of DNA methylation and hydroxymethylation in mammalian development. *Curr Topics Devel Biol.* 2013;104:47-83.

38. Wen L, Tang F. Genomic distribution and possible functions of DNA hydroxymethylation in the brain. *Genomics.* 2014;104(5):341-6.

39. Santiago M, Antunes C, Guedes M, Sousa N, Marques CJ. TET enzymes and DNA hydroxymethylation in neural development and function – How critical are they? *Genomics*. 2014;104(5):334-40.

40. Feil R, Fraga MF. Epigenetics and the environment: Emerging patterns and implications. *Nat Rev Genet*. 2011;13(2):97-109.

41. Maleszka R. Epigenetic integration of environmental and genomic signals in honey bees. *Epigenetics*. 2008;3(4):188-92.

42. Kucharski R, Maleszka J, Foret S, Maleszka R. Nutritional control of reproductive status in honeybees via DNA methylation. *Science*. 2008;319(5871):1827-30.

43. Waterland RA, Jirtle RL. Transposable elements: Targets for early nutritional effects on epigenetic gene regulation. *Mol Cell Biol*. 2003;23(15):5293-300.

44. Lillycrop KA, Phillips ES, Jackson AA, Hanson MA, Burdge GC. Dietary protein restriction of pregnant rats induces and folic acid supplementation prevents epigenetic modification of hepatic gene expression in the offspring. *J Nutr*. 2005;135(6):1382-6.

45. Lillycrop KA, Slater-Jefferies JL, Hanson MA, Godfrey KM, Jackson AA, Burdge GC. Induction of altered epigenetic regulation of the hepatic glucocorticoid receptor in the offspring of rats fed a protein-restricted diet during pregnancy suggests that reduced DNA methyltransferase-1 expression is involved in impaired DNA methylation and changes in histone modifications. *Br J Nutr*. 2007;97(6):1064-73.

46. Burdge GC, Phillips ES, Dunn RL, Jackson AA, Lillycrop KA. Effect of reduced maternal protein consumption during pregnancy in the rat on plasma lipid concentrations and expression of peroxisomal proliferator-activated receptors in the liver and adipose tissue of the offspring. *Nutr Res*. 2004;24(8):639-46.

47. Gluckman PD, Lillycrop KA, Vickers MH, Pleasants AB, Phillips ES, Beedle AS, et al. Metabolic plasticity during mammalian development is directionally dependent on early nutritional status. *Proc Natl Acad Sci U S A*. 2007;104(31):12796-800.

48. Gluckman PD, Hanson MA, Spencer HG. Predictive adaptive responses and human evolution. *Trends Ecol Evol*. 2005;20(10):527-33.

49. Vucetic Z, Kimmel J, Totoki K, Hollenbeck E, Reyes TM. Maternal high-fat diet alters methylation and gene expression of dopamine and opioid-related genes. *Endocrinology*. 2010;151(10):4756-64.

50. Tobi EW, Lumey LH, Talens RP, Kremer D, Putter H, Stein AD, et al. DNA methylation differences after exposure to prenatal famine are common and timing- and sex-specific. *Hum Mol Genet*. 2009;18(21):4046-53.

51. Steegers-Theunissen RP, Obermann-Borst SA, Kremer D, Lindemans J, Siebel C, Steegers EA, et al. Periconceptional maternal folic acid use of 400 microg per day is related to increased methylation of the IGF2 gene in the very young child. *PloS One*. 2009;4(11):e7845.

52. Jacobsen SC, Brons C, Bork-Jensen J, Ribel-Madsen R, Yang B, Lara E, et al. Effects of short-term high-fat overfeeding on genome-wide DNA methylation in the skeletal muscle of healthy young men. *Diabetologia*. 2012;55(12):3341-9.

53. Gao X, Jia M, Zhang Y, Breitling LP, Brenner H. DNA methylation changes of whole blood cells in response to active smoking exposure in adults: A systematic review of DNA methylation studies. *Clin Epigenet*. 2015;7:113.

54. Hannum G, Guinney J, Zhao L, Zhang L, Hughes G, Sadda S, et al. Genome-wide methylation profiles reveal quantitative views of human aging rates. *Molec Cell*. 2013;49(2):359-67.

55. Horvath S. DNA methylation age of human tissues and cell types. *Genome Biol*. 2013;14(10):R115.

56. Zhang Y, Wilson R, Heiss J, Breitling LP, Saum KU, Schottker B, et al. DNA methylation signatures in peripheral blood strongly predict all-cause mortality. *Nat Comm*. 2017;8:14617.

57. Marioni RE, Shah S, McRae AF, Chen BH, Colicino E, Harris SE, et al. DNA methylation age of blood predicts all-cause mortality in later life. *Genome Biol*. 2015;16:25.

58. Godfrey KM, Sheppard A, Gluckman PD, Lillycrop KA, Burdge GC, McLean C, et al. Epigenetic gene promoter methylation at birth is associated with child's later adiposity. *Diabetes*. 2011;60(5):1528-34.

59. Clarke-Harris R, Wilkin TJ, Hosking J, Pinkney J, Jeffery AN, Metcalf BS, et al. PGC1alpha promoter methylation in blood at 5-7 years predicts adiposity from 9 to 14 years (EarlyBird 50). *Diabetes*. 2014;63(7):2528-37.

8

Epigenetic mechanisms in bone development

ELIZABETH M CURTIS, NICHOLAS C HARVEY
AND CYRUS COOPER

INTRODUCTION

As documented in Chapter 7, epigenetic mechanisms provide a potential explanation for observed associations between early environmental exposures and later health and disease through modulation of gene expression. Evidence that such processes may be important in long-term skeletal health is now emerging from unique cohorts such as the Southampton Women's Survey, in which a well-established discovery pipeline has identified methylation marks at genes implicated in vitamin D metabolism and cell senescence, which are associated with later bone outcomes (1).

VITAMIN D AND DNA METHYLATION

Vitamin D has been shown to be an environmental factor which may play an important role in bone development from the fetal period onwards, perhaps through regulation of DNA methylation. In terms of a mechanistic link between maternal vitamin D status and offspring bone mass, data suggest that this may be mediated, at least in part, through placental calcium transport (2). More recent research has suggested that placental amino acid transport might also be partly regulated by maternal 25(OH)-vitamin D [25(OH)D] status and vitamin D binding protein levels, presenting another complementary mechanism for this association (3). In the Southampton Women's Survey, mRNA expression of an active ATP-dependent placental calcium transporter, PMCA3, in placental tissue, was positively associated with offspring bone area and bone mineral content of the whole body site at birth (4). The regulation of placental calcium transfer is poorly characterized in humans, and any mechanistic role of vitamin D remains to be elucidated, but members of the PMCA family appear to be regulated by $1,25(OH)_2$-vitamin D [$1,25(OH)_2D$] in animal studies (5). Further insights into vitamin D metabolism indicate that the 1α-hydroxylase gene is regulated by $1,25(OH)_2D$, through vitamin D receptor (VDR)-mediated transcriptional regulation. Furthermore, the ongoing regulation of vitamin D metabolism may involve methylation of sites in the 1α-hydroxylase promoter region, with the $1,25(OH)_2$-vitamin D/VDR/RXR complex inducing DNA methylation at the *1α-hydroxylase* promoter, while parathyroid hormone (PTH) signalling leads to demethylation of this region through a different pathway. This suggests a role for epigenetic processes in the vitamin D–parathyroid hormone axis (6,7).

Collection of umbilical cord samples from the Princess Anne Hospital Cohort and the Southampton Women's Survey has allowed the elucidation of relationships between epigenetic marking at candidate sites, identified through array approaches (8), and offspring bone size, mineralization and density. An example of a pipeline for identification of methyl marks from epigenome wide to candidate is summarised in Figure 8.1 (1).

In 66 mother-offspring pairs from the Princess Anne Hospital Cohort study, percentage methylation at 2 CpG sites in the promoter region of endothelial nitric oxide synthase (*eNOS*) in umbilical cord was positively related to the child's whole body bone area, bone mineral content and areal bone mineral density at age nine years (r = 0.28 to 0.34, p = 0.005 to 0.02) (9). eNOS has been shown to play a mechanistic role in the function of osteoblasts, osteocytes and osteoclasts, and there has been evidence of a positive effect of nitrate use on bone density in clinical populations (10–13).

In the Southampton Women's Survey, greater methylation at four out of six CpG sites in the promoter region of retinoid X receptor-alpha (*RXRA*) in umbilical cord was correlated with lower offspring BMC corrected for body size at 4 years old, as shown in Figure 8.2 (β = −2.1 to −3.4 g/sd, p = 0.002 to 0.047), with the results supported by findings from a second independent cohort, the Princess Anne Hospital Study (14). In this study, an estimate of maternal free vitamin D index was inversely related to *RXRA* methylation at CpG 4/5 (chromosome 9, 136355593, 600+). As previously stated, RXRA forms a heterodimer with several nuclear hormones known to influence bone metabolism, including $1,25(OH)_2$-vitamin D, perhaps implying that maternal 25(OH)D status might play a permissive role in the transcriptional regulation of the *RXRA* gene. Evidence of functional significance was obtained through altered response to transcription factor binding and further characterization of these processes is ongoing, but clearly replication in independent cohorts will be required to validate such findings.

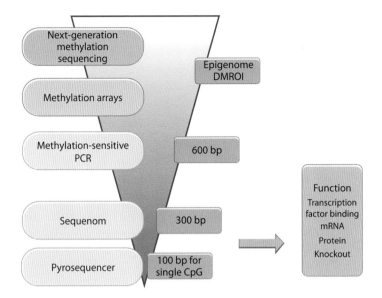

Figure 8.1 Schematic representation of the investigation of methyl marking from epigenome to candidate. Next-generation methylation sequencing allows identification of individual methyl marks across the entire methylome. Array-based approaches permit identification of differentially methylated regions of interest (DMROI) across a wide genomic area – commonly used '450k' methylation arrays assess methylation at 450,000 CpG sites throughout the genome, but '850k' arrays offering wider coverage are now available. Refinement of candidate selection and investigation of individual CpG methylation may be obtained from techniques such as Sequenom and pyrosequencing, through which methylation can be measured at the individual CpG level. Functional significance may be elucidated from transcription factor binding, mRNA and protein expression, and further validated using knockout models in cell lines and whole animals. (Adapted with permission from Harvey NC et al. *J Bone Miner Res.* 2014;29(9):1917-25.)

Associations between maternal 25(OH)D status and *RXRA* methylation could be mediated by a variety of mechanisms. Studies have shown that vitamin D may interact with the epigenome on multiple levels. The critical genes in the vitamin D signalling system, including those coding for VDR and the enzymes 25-hydroxylase (CYP2R1), 1α-hydroxylase (CYP27B1) and 24-hydroxylase (CYP24A1) have large CpG islands in their promoter regions and therefore can be silenced by DNA methylation. Second, the VDR/RXR heterodimer has been shown to physically interact with proteins that are able to remodel the chromatin environment through coactivator and corepressor proteins, which in turn are in contact with histone modifiers, such as histone acetyltransferases (HATs), histone deacetylases (HDACs), histone methyltransferases (HMTs) and with chromatin remodelers. Thirdly, a number of genes encoding for chromatin modifiers and remodelers are primary targets of VDR and its ligands, and finally, there is evidence that certain VDR ligands have DNA demethylating effects (15).

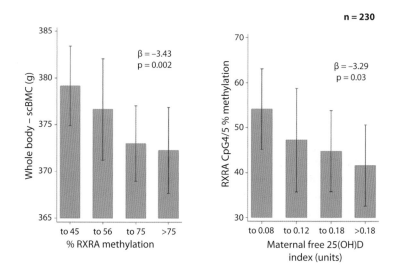

Figure 8.2 Relationships between percent methylation at the RXRA promoter and BMC corrected for whole body size (left), and the association between maternal free 25(OH)D index and RXRA methylation at CpG 4/5 (right), n = 230, in Southampton Women's Survey. (Reproduced with permission from Harvey NC et al. *J Bone Miner Res.* 2014;29(3):600-7.)

It is possible that a greater understanding of the actions of vitamin D on DNA methylation may come from EWAS studies. An EWAS analysis of DNA methylation in severely vitamin D deficient African American adolescents demonstrated altered methylation in several genes, including genes involved in vitamin D metabolism such as the 24 and 25-hydroxylase genes (16). Other studies have assessed the DNA methylation in CYP enzymes which are part of the vitamin D metabolism pathway and found a relationship between methylation of the genes *CYP2R1* (25-hydroxylase) and *CYP24A1 (24-hydroxylase)* and variations in circulating 25(OH)D levels (7). Another study, using the ALSPAC cohort and the Norwegian Mother and Child Cohort (MoBa) demonstrated no convincing associations between maternal 25(OH)D status and DNA methylation in the umbilical cord blood of 1416 newborn babies using 450k array analysis, thereby covering 473,731CpG DNA methylation sites (17). The authors suggested that to further identify associations, larger consortium studies, expanded genomic coverage and investigation of alternative cell types or 25(OH)D status at different gestational time points was needed.

DNA METHYLATION, AND SKELETAL DEVELOPMENT AND HOMEOSTASIS

Previous array analysis of umbilical cord samples from the Princess Anne Hospital Cohort and the Southampton Women's Survey (8) identified an association between offspring fat mass and methylation at another locus, *CDKN2A* (8,18,19).

The *CDKN2A* locus encodes two cell cycle inhibitors: p14^ARF and P16^INK4a, which play roles in cellular senescence and ageing. The *CDKN2A* locus also encodes the long non-coding RNA ANRIL (antisense non-coding RNA in the *INK4* locus), a 3834bp transcript which can negatively regulate *p16INK4a*. SNPs within the *CDKN2A* locus, particularly those located within *ANRIL*, have been associated with cardiovascular disease, diabetes and frailty (20), and DNA methylation at this locus has recently been demonstrated to vary with age (21).

Studies have demonstrated links between perinatal *CDKN2A* methylation and offspring fat mass, demonstrating it is a marker for later adiposity (22). The functional relationships between fat and bone are well characterised, and mediated via both mechanical and endocrine pathways (23). Furthermore, DNA methylation at CpG sites within the *CDKN2A* gene was associated with offspring bone mass at age 4 and 6 (24) (Figure 8.3).

Such work emphasises the importance of DNA methylation in epigenetic processes in bone metabolism, particularly with regard to loci implicated in cellular differentiation, cell cycle regulation and bone cell function, from early in development to older age.

EPIGENETIC MECHANISMS IN DEVELOPMENT AND SENESCENCE

In bone development, DNA methylation has been shown to play an important role in osteoblast differentiation; one study demonstrated transitional hypomethylation of several genes, including *RUNX2*, *osteocalcin* and *CDKN2A* in bone marrow stromal cells in their differentiation towards an osteoblastic lineage (25). Another study identified the importance of cyclin-dependent kinases and their inhibitors in this process – in the osteogenic differentiation of adipose-derived mesenchymal stem cells, the promoters of *RUNX2*, *osteocalcin* and *osterix* genes are actively demethylated in a process dependent upon growth arrest and DNA-damage-inducible protein, GADD45, which is known to interact with both *CDK1* and *CDKN1A* (26,27). Wnt 3a has also been shown to play a role in osteoblast differentiation through stimulation of bone morphogenetic protein 2 (*BMP2*) and alkaline phosphatase (*ALP*) expression, in a process which appears to be regulated by *BMP2* and *ALP* promoter methylation (28).

In differentiated bone tissue of various cell types, the importance of DNA methylation marks has been demonstrated in bone remodelling and osteoclastogenesis through regulation of the receptor activator of nuclear factor NFκB ligand (*RANKL*) gene and its soluble decoy receptor osteoprotegerin (*OPG*) (29). Finally, DNA methylation has been shown play a role in the ultimate state of osteoblast differentiation to osteocytes embedded in mineralised bone, through the regulation of various genes including *ALP* and *sclerostin* (*SOST*) (30–32), and through the transduction of mechanical stimuli (33).

At the other end of the lifecourse, the relevance of DNA methylation has been shown in the pathogenesis of osteoporosis; it has been demonstrated that hypomethylation of *Alu* elements, (interspersed repetitive DNA elements) are associated with lower bone mineral density in postmenopausal women (34). In another

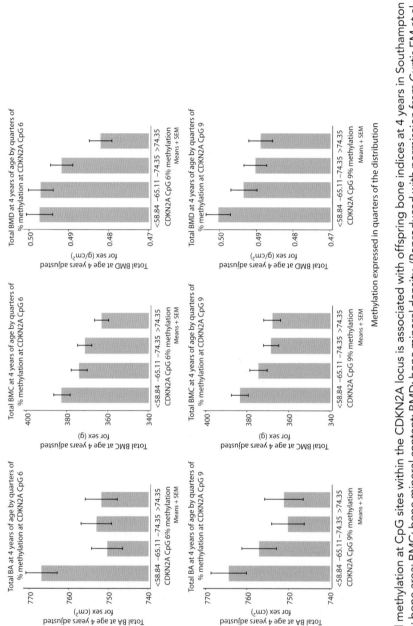

Figure 8.3 Perinatal methylation at CpG sites within the CDKN2A locus is associated with offspring bone indices at 4 years in Southampton Women's Survey. BA: bone area; BMC: bone mineral content; BMD: bone mineral density. (Reproduced with permission from Curtis EM et al. *J Bone Miner Res.* 2017; 32(10):2030-40.)

study, methylation of *SOST* in blood samples was increased in osteoporotic patients, and SOST mRNA in bone cells decreased, in a suggested compensatory mechanism in osteoporosis in order to promote bone formation (35).

Genome-wide methylation profiling studies in older patients comparing individuals with low versus normal BMD have also suggested early life influences on bone quality in older age. One study, comparing bone biopsies of older people with hip fractures to osteoarthritis patients, identified differentially methylated regions (DMRs) enriched in genes associated with cell differentiation and skeletal embryogenesis, including those in the *homeobox* superfamily, which suggests the existence of a developmental component in the predisposition to osteoporosis. Genes encoding the cyclin-dependent kinase inhibitor *CKDN1C* (known to be regulated by the vitamin D receptor) and cyclin-dependent kinase *CDK20* were both differentially methylated in osteoporosis versus osteoarthritis samples (36). A multiomics analysis incorporating gene expression, DNA methylation and miRNA data in high BMD versus low BMD women identified four potential regulatory patterns of gene expression to influence BMD status, two of which – the mTOR and insulin signalling pathway – have been linked to bone cell differentiation and postnatal bone growth (37).

Therefore, there is evidence that DNA methylation at loci important for cell cycle regulation, differentiation and function of bone cells can have an impact on bone development and bone health throughout life.

VALIDATION AND FUNCTIONAL RELEVANCE OF EPIGENETIC SIGNALS

From the studies described, it is apparent that epigenetic marking in early life is associated with later phenotypic variation. However, given the potential tissue specificity of epigenetic signals, the variation of such marks over time and the difficulty in differentiating cause from effect, the exact characterization of epigenetic mechanisms in disease etiology and pathology is a very complex process (38,39). Epigenetic marks identified in human cohorts through array and candidate investigation must be replicated in separate independent cohorts to robustly establish associations with later disease. However, a large EWAS, assessing the association of up to 473,882 CpGs quantified in whole blood with BMD in 4614 North American and European adults, in a discovery cohort, and 901 in a replication cohort failed to find any substantial methylation-bone relationships using the Infinium Human Methylation 450 BeadChip (40). Cell heterogeneity in whole blood may be a limiting factor here – indeed, targeted EWAS in specific cell types in blood with a clear role in bone biology, that is, monocytes due to their role in osteoclastogenesis, may be more fruitful.

Experimental work using cell culture and animal models is also required to document the detailed molecular processes, regulation and functional consequences. A combination of such fundamental investigation and linkage to disease development will be essential to fully understand the role of epigenetic mechanisms in the development of osteoporosis. In the meantime, whether the observed epigenetic marks are cause or consequence, if replicated, such signals may well present useful novel biomarkers for later adverse bone development.

REFERENCES

1. Harvey N, Dennison E, Cooper C. Osteoporosis: A lifecourse approach. *J Bone Miner Res.* 2014;29(9):1917-25.
2. Javaid MK, Crozier SR, Harvey NC, Gale CR, Dennison EM, Boucher BJ, et al. Maternal vitamin D status during pregnancy and childhood bone mass at age 9 years: A longitudinal study. *Lancet.* 2006;367(9504):36-43.
3. Cleal JK, Day PE, Simner CL, Barton SJ, Mahon PA, Inskip HM, et al. Placental amino acid transport may be regulated by maternal vitamin D and vitamin D-binding protein: Results from the Southampton Women's Survey. *Br J Nutr.* 2015;113(12):1903-10.
4. Martin R, Harvey NC, Crozier SR, Poole JR, Javaid MK, Dennison EM, et al. Placental calcium transporter (PMCA3) gene expression predicts intrauterine bone mineral accrual. *Bone.* 2007;40(5):1203-8.
5. Kip SN, Strehler EE. Vitamin D3 upregulates plasma membrane Ca2+-ATPase expression and potentiates apico-basal Ca2+ flux in MDCK cells. *Am J Physiol Renal Physiol.* 2004;286(2):F363-F9.
6. Takeyama K, Kato S. The vitamin D3 1alpha-hydroxylase gene and its regulation by active vitamin D3. *Biosci Biotechnol Biochem.* 2011;75 (2):208-13.
7. Zhou Y, Zhao LJ, Xu X, Ye A, Travers-Gustafson D, Zhou B, et al. DNA methylation levels of CYP2R1 and CYP24A1 predict vitamin D response variation. *J Steroid Biochem Mol Biol.* 2014;144PA:207-14.
8. Godfrey KM, Sheppard A, Gluckman PD, Lillycrop KA, Burdge GC, McLean C, et al. Epigenetic gene promoter methylation at birth is associated with child's later adiposity. *Diabetes.* 2011;60(5):1528-34.
9. Harvey NC, Lillycrop KA, Garratt E, Sheppard A, McLean C, Burdge G, et al. Evaluation of methylation status of the eNOS promoter at birth in relation to childhood bone mineral content. *Calcif Tissue Int.* 2012;90(2):120-7.
10. Zaman G, Pitsillides AA, Rawlinson SC, Suswillo RF, Mosley JR, Cheng MZ, et al. Mechanical strain stimulates nitric oxide production by rapid activation of endothelial nitric oxide synthase in osteocytes. *J Bone Miner Res.* 1999;14(7):1123-31.
11. Sabanai K, Tsutsui M, Sakai A, Hirasawa H, Tanaka S, Nakamura E, et al. Genetic disruption of all NO synthase isoforms enhances BMD and bone turnover in mice in vivo: Involvement of the renin-angiotensin system. *J Bone Miner Res.* 2008;23(5):633-43.
12. Nilforoushan D, Gramoun A, Glogauer M, Manolson MF. Nitric oxide enhances osteoclastogenesis possibly by mediating cell fusion. *Nitric Oxide.* 2009;21(1):27-36.
13. Jamal SA, Browner WS, Bauer DC, Cummings SR. Intermittent use of nitrates increases bone mineral density: The study of osteoporotic fractures. *J Bone Miner Res.* 1998;13(11):1755-9.
14. Harvey NC, Sheppard A, Godfrey KM, McLean C, Garratt E, Ntani G, et al. Childhood bone mineral content is associated with methylation status of the RXRA promoter at birth. *J Bone Miner Res.* 2014;29(3):600-7.

15. Fetahu IS, Höbaus J, Kállay E. Vitamin D and the epigenome. *Frontiers Physiol.* 2014;5(164):1-12.

16. Zhu H, Wang X, Shi H, Su S, Harshfield GA, Gutin B, et al. A genome-wide methylation study of severe vitamin D deficiency in African American adolescents. *J Pediatr.* 2013;162(5):1004-9.e1.

17. Suderman M, Stene LC, Bohlin J, Page CM, Holvik K, Parr CL, et al. 25-Hydroxyvitamin D in pregnancy and genome wide cord blood DNA methylation in two pregnancy cohorts (MoBa and ALSPAC). *J Steroid Biochem Molec Biol.* 2016;159:102-9.

18. Lillycrop KA MR, Teh AL, Cheong CY, Dogra S, Clarke-Harris R, Barton S, et al. 8th World Congress on Developmental Origins of Health and Disease. *J Devel Origins Health Disease.* 2013;4(s2):S1509 DOI: 10.017/S2040174413000421.

19. Murray R, Bryant J, Titcombe P, Barton SJ, Inskip H, Harvey NC, et al. DNA methylation at birth within the promoter of ANRIL predicts markers of cardiovascular risk at 9 years. *Clin Epigenetics.* 2016;8:90.

20. Congrains A, Kamide K, Oguro R, Yasuda O, Miyata K, Yamamoto E, et al. Genetic variants at the 9p21 locus contribute to atherosclerosis through modulation of ANRIL and CDKN2A/B. *Atherosclerosis.* 2012;220(2):449-55.

21. Bell CG, Xia Y, Yuan W, Gao F, Ward K, Roos L, et al. Novel regional age-associated DNA methylation changes within human common disease-associated loci. *Genome Biol.* 2016;17(1):193.

22. Lillycrop K, Murray R, Cheong C, Teh AL, Clarke-Harris R, Barton S, et al. ANRIL promoter DNA methylation: A perinatal marker for later adiposity. *EBioMedicine.* 2017;19:60-72.

23. Johansson H, Kanis JA, Oden A, McCloskey E, Chapurlat RD, Christiansen C, et al. A meta-analysis of the association of fracture risk and body mass index in women. *J Bone Miner Res.* 2014;29(1):223-33.

24. Curtis EM, Murray R, Titcombe P, Cook E, Clarke-Harris R, Costello P, et al. Perinatal DNA methylation at CDKN2A is associated with offspring bone mass: Findings from the Southampton Women's Survey. *J Bone Miner Res.* 2017;32(10):2030-40.

25. Kang MI, Kim HS, Jung YC, Kim YH, Hong SJ, Kim MK, et al. Transitional CpG methylation between promoters and retroelements of tissue-specific genes during human mesenchymal cell differentiation. *J Cell Biochem.* 2007;102(1):224-39.

26. Zhang RP, Shao JZ, Xiang LX. GADD45A protein plays an essential role in active DNA demethylation during terminal osteogenic differentiation of adipose-derived mesenchymal stem cells. *J Biol Chem.* 2011;286(47):41083-94.

27. Ghayor C, Weber FE. Epigenetic regulation of bone remodeling and its impacts in osteoporosis. *Int J Mol Sci.* 2016;17(9).

28. Cho YD, Yoon WJ, Kim WJ, Woo KM, Baek JH, Lee G, et al. Epigenetic modifications and canonical wingless/int-1 class (WNT) signaling enable trans-differentiation of nonosteogenic cells into osteoblasts. *J Cell Biochem.* 2014;289(29):20120-8.

29. Delgado-Calle J, Sañudo C, Fernández AF, García-Renedo R, Fraga MF, Riancho JA. Role of DNA methylation in the regulation of the RANKL-OPG system in human bone. *Epigenetics*. 2012;7(1):83-91.

30. Delgado-Calle J, Riancho J. The role of DNA methylation in common skeletal disorders. *Biology*. 2012;1(3):698.

31. Delgado-Calle J, Sanudo C, Bolado A, Fernandez AF, Arozamena J, Pascual-Carra MA, et al. DNA methylation contributes to the regulation of sclerostin expression in human osteocytes. *J Bone Miner Res*. 2012;27(4):926-37.

32. Delgado-Calle J, Sanudo C, Sanchez-Verde L, Garcia-Renedo RJ, Arozamena J, Riancho JA. Epigenetic regulation of alkaline phosphatase in human cells of the osteoblastic lineage. *Bone*. 2011;49(4):830-8.

33. Hupkes M, van Someren EP, Middelkamp SH, Piek E, van Zoelen EJ, Dechering KJ. DNA methylation restricts spontaneous multi-lineage differentiation of mesenchymal progenitor cells, but is stable during growth factor-induced terminal differentiation. *Biochim Biophys Acta* 2011;1813(5):839-49.

34. Jintaridth P, Tungtrongchitr R, Preutthipan S, Mutirangura A. Hypomethylation of Alu elements in post-menopausal women with osteoporosis. *PloS One*. 2013;8(8):e70386.

35. Reppe S, Noer A, Grimholt RM, Halldorsson BV, Medina-Gomez C, Gautvik VT, et al. Methylation of bone SOST, its mRNA, and serum sclerostin levels correlate strongly with fracture risk in postmenopausal women. *J Bone Miner Res*. 2015;30(2):249-56.

36. Delgado-Calle J, Fernandez AF, Sainz J, Zarrabeitia MT, Sanudo C, Garcia-Renedo R, et al. Genome-wide profiling of bone reveals differentially methylated regions in osteoporosis and osteoarthritis. *Arthritis Rheum*. 2013;65(1):197-205.

37. Zhang JG, Tan LJ, Xu C, He H, Tian Q, Zhou Y, et al. Integrative analysis of transcriptomic and epigenomic data to reveal regulation patterns for BMD variation. *PloS One*. 2015;10(9):e0138524.

38. Hanson M, Godfrey KM, Lillycrop KA, Burdge GC, Gluckman PD. Developmental plasticity and developmental origins of non-communicable disease: Theoretical considerations and epigenetic mechanisms. *Prog Biophys Mol Biol*. 2011;106(1):272-80.

39. Xie M, Hong C, Zhang B, Lowdon RF, Xing X, Li D, et al. DNA hypomethylation within specific transposable element families associates with tissue-specific enhancer landscape. *Nat Genet*. 2013;45(7):836-41.

40. Morris JA, Tsai PC, Joehanes R, Zheng J, Trajanoska K, Soerensen M, et al. Epigenome-wide association of DNA methylation in whole blood with bone mineral density. *J Bone Miner Res*. 2017;32(8):1644-50.

9

The material and structural basis of the growth-related gain and age-related loss of bone strength

EGO SEEMAN

INTRODUCTION

Differences in bone size, shape, microstructure and material composition account for differences in bone strength between individuals, sexes and races. The variance in bone morphology is established during the first 2 years of life and does not vary much subsequently. An individual's bone traits may occupy different percentile locations but whatever that percentile, the trait tracks from early infancy through adolescence to adulthood in the same trajectory whether this ranking is the 95th, 50th or 5th percentile.

During growth, an increasing volume of bone matrix is assembled with varying medullary and cortical canal void volumes establishing bone's external dimension and differing configuration of its matrix forming the compact bone (the least porous compartment), the transitional compartment and the most porous trabecular compartment. Bone size is achieved using relatively more void than matrix volume, so larger bones are assembled with relatively less material; larger bones have a lower volumetric apparent bone mineral density (BMD). Smaller bones are more robustly assembled. Asians have long bones with thicker cortices relative to their cross-sectional size, less porous cortices with a higher matrix mineral density than Caucasians. Sex and racial differences in bone dimensions and microstructure become most evident at puberty, partly due to differences in pubertal age. Later puberty in males than females, or Caucasians than Asians, results in greater appendicular dimensions in males than females and Caucasians than Asians because the longer prepubertal years of the more rapid appendicular than axial growth. Longer intrapubertal growth confers greater axial length in males than females but comparable axial length in Caucasians and Asians.

At the onset of adulthood, completion of longitudinal growth is associated with slowing of periosteal apposition. Remodelling upon the intracortical, endocortical and trabecular components of bone's internal (endosteal) surface continues slowly and maintains bone's material composition by replacing old or damaged bone with an equal volume of new bone so that no permanent structural deterioration occurs.

Around midlife, remodelling becomes unbalanced in both sexes and all races, and becomes rapid after menopause, accelerating structural deterioration in females more than in males. The surface area/matrix volume configuration of the skeleton established during growth by modelling and remodelling partly determines the accessibility of bone matrix to being remodelled during adulthood; higher remodelling during growth assembles a more porous bone with a larger surface area/volume configuration in adulthood which is more vulnerable to being deteriorated when rapid unbalanced remodelling emerges after menopause. Trabecular bone, with its higher surface area/volume configuration, is more readily remodelled and lost than cortical bone. Trabecular bone loss is self-limiting because trabeculae perforate and disappear. A more robustly assembled structure with a smaller surface area/matrix volume, as found in Asians, is less accessible to being remodelled, enabling slower structural deterioration during advancing age when remodelling becomes unbalanced.

Variances in bone traits achieved during growth are greater than rates of bone loss during aging so that attention to factors influencing peak bone structure during the first two decades of life are important but bone loss becomes increasingly important as age advances. Trabeculae disappear and intracortical porosity increases the intracortical surface area making cortical bone, 80% of the skeleton, the source of 70% of all bone loss. Cortical bone loss is self-perpetuating, as more remodelling creates more surface upon which unbalanced remodelling can be initiated; a diminishing total bone volume is lost ever more rapidly, predisposing to fragility fractures in advanced age.

INTRAUTERINE AND POSTNATAL GROWTH: TRAIT VARIANCES ARE ESTABLISHED EARLY

The variance of bone traits like bone mass is large: 1 standard deviation (SD) is about 10% to 15% of the mean (1). Thus individuals at the 95th and 5th percentiles for bone size differ by ~50% in that trait. The variance in the rate of bone loss in adulthood is about an order of magnitude less (1 SD = 1% of the mean). Consequently, the difference in the percentile location of a trait at the completion of growth is an important determinant of bone strength and fracture risk in advanced age (2). Differences in bone structure appear during intrauterine life, but at least for femur length determined using ultrasound imaging, there is no evidence that ranking in a given percentile is established in utero. On the contrary, the location of an individual's femur length in a given quartile varies throughout gestation such that under 10% of individuals have femur length at birth in the same quartile as found in earlier stages of gestation (3) (Figure 9.1).

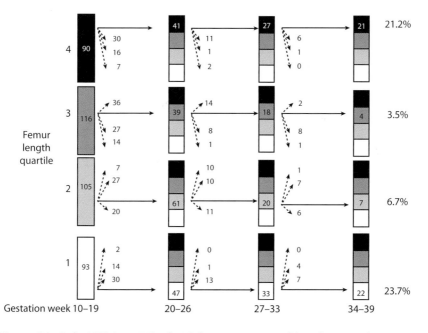

Figure 9.1 Only 13% (n = 54) of 412 femurs measured by ultrasound in utero remained within the same quartile during gestation. Numbers on the right refer to the percentage tracking within a given quartile. The numbers to the right of the bars give of the disposition of individuals' femur length from their baseline quartile location through gestation. The numbers are fetuses that kept their quartile (solid array) or deviated (dashed line) from quartile 1 (white), quartile 2 (light grey), quartile 3 (dark grey) and quartile 4 (black). (Adapted with permission from Bjornerem A et al. *J Bone Miner Res*. 2010;25(5):1029-33.)

INFANCY AND CHILDHOOD GROWTH

Some studies report associations between bone traits at birth and adulthood (4,5). For example, crown–heel length (CHL) at 6 months or later, but not at birth, predicted height, bone size, mass and strength almost two decades later (6,7). CHL or height tracked from 6 months of age through childhood and adolescence to adulthood. This also applied to total and regional bone mass and size, tibial and radial cross-sectional area and indices of bending and compressive strength first measured at 11.5 years of age and then measured during the subsequent 7 years to 18 years of age. Bone traits also track through puberty without change in percentile location. Loro et al. report that the percentile ranking of traits at Tanner stage 2 was unchanged during 3 years, and 60% to 90% of the variance at maturity was accounted for by variance before puberty (8). An individual with a larger vertebral or femoral shaft cross-section or higher vertebral volumetric (vBMD) or femoral cortical area than their peers before puberty retained this relative position to maturity. Premenopausal daughters of women with fractures have structural abnormalities at the corresponding site, suggesting that familial resemblance of bone traits at maturity are established during growth (9).

Bone modelling assembles bone size and its shape according to a genetic programme; fetal limb buds grown in vitro develop the shape of the proximal femur (10). Nevertheless, environmental factors influence bone morphology. Differences in bone size in the playing arm and non-playing arm of tennis players attest to the ability of periosteal apposition to model bone in response to loading during growth (11); comparable effects in adulthood are not reported.

In prepubertal girls, tibial cross-sectional shape is already elliptical at 10 years of age (12). During 2 years, periosteal apposition increased ellipticity by adding twice the amount of bone anteriorly and posteriorly as medially and laterally (Figure 9.2). Consequently, estimates of bending strength increase more in the antero-posterior than mediolateral direction. Greater periosteal apposition on the anterior and posterior surfaces than on the medial and lateral surfaces creates the elliptical shape of the tibia and demonstrates how strength is optimized while mass is minimized by modelling and remodelling being point-specific. Modifying the spatial distribution of the bone material rather than using more material is energy saving. If cortical thickness increased by the same amount of periosteal apposition at each point around the perimeter of a cross-section, the amount of bone producing the same increase in bending resistance would be fourfold more than observed.

This is further illustrated by the heterogeneity in femoral neck shape (13). At the junction with the shaft, femoral neck (FN) size and ellipticity is greatest. Size decreases and then increases, and the cross-section becomes more circular. This diversity in total cross-sectional size and shape from cross-sectional slice to cross-sectional slice is achieved using a similar amount of material. The constant amount of material is distributed differently in space with different proportions of void volume at each cross-section. The same amount of bone is assembled as a larger cross-section with mainly cortical bone adjacent to the femoral shaft, and most of this distributed inferiorly. More proximally, the proportion of bone that is cortical decreases while the proportion that is trabecular increases reciprocally.

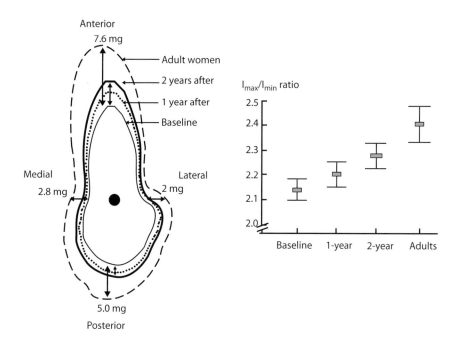

Figure 9.2 Distribution of mass around the tibia. Focal periosteal apposition varied at each degree around the bone perimeter. More bone was deposited at the anterio-posterior (AP) regions than at the mediolateral (ML) regions, increasing the ellipticity and bending strength more along the AP axis (I_{max}) than the ML axis (I_{min}). (Adapted with permission from Wang Q et al. *J Clin Endocrinol Metab*. 2009;94(5):1555-61.)

Cortices become thinner, and at the femoral head junction, most bone is trabecular and the cortex is thin and evenly distributed around the perimeter. Differing periosteal apposition at each point around the bone perimeter is accompanied by concurrent resorption on the endosteal surfaces of the bone. In tubular bones lightness is achieved by endocortical resorption, which excavates the marrow cavity, shifting the thickening cortex outwards, distant from the neutral axis, increasing the bone's resistance to bending (14). Wang et al. reported that the amount of bone deposited during 2 years on the periosteal surface in prepubertal children with larger tibial cross-sections was no different to the amount deposited on the periosteal surface of smaller cross-sections (12).

Thus, larger bones deposit *less* bone *relative* to their starting cross-sectional size than smaller bones because resistance to bending requires less material be deposited upon the periosteal surface of a larger than smaller bone. Lightness is also achieved in larger bones by making them more porous, and the matrix less completely mineralised. Larger bones also excavate a larger medullary canal by higher rates of modelling-based endocortical resorption, so larger bones are relatively lighter. Larger bones also have higher cortical porosity (15) (Figure 9.3). Both features result in bones with a lower apparent vBMD.

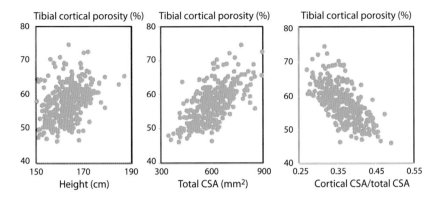

Figure 9.3 The greater the height and total cross-sectional area of the tibia, the higher the cortical porosity (left and middle panels). The larger the cortical area as a proportion of the total tibial cross-sectional area (and so the smaller the medullary area), the lower the porosity. CSA, cross-sectional area. (Adapted with permission from Bjornerem A et al. *J Bone Miner Res.* 2013;28(9):2017-26.)

Individuals with smaller tubular bone cross-sections assemble them with *more* mass relative to their size, forming a bone with a higher apparent vBMD. In bones with a smaller cross-section, the liability to fracture due to slenderness is offset by more periosteal apposition relative to their starting cross-sectional size, and excavation of a smaller medullary canal and lower cortical porosity so vBMD is higher. Asians have smaller bones with a lower cortical porosity and higher vBMD than Caucasians (16). So, a high peak vBMD is *not* the result of increased bone formation (mass has a high energy cost), it is the result of *reduced* bone resorption. (The resorption is not followed by formation and is a modelling, not remodelling.) Similarly, a lower vBMD is the result of more bone resorption, not less bone formation.

PUBERTY AND SEX DIFFERENCES IN MORPHOLOGY

Growth in height is the result of appendicular and axial growth (17). Appendicular and axial groups are rapid at birth and slow precipitously after birth. Around 1 year of age, appendicular growth velocity accelerates and remains about twice that of axial growth velocity until puberty, so most of the growth in height before puberty is due to growth of the legs. At puberty, appendicular growth decelerates while axial growth accelerates. Sex differences in bone length, width, mass, and strength emerge largely during puberty. During the first 2 years of puberty (11–13 years in girls and 13–15 years in boys) the contribution of axial and appendicular growth to the standing height is similar (7.7 vs 7.4 cm in girls and 8.5 vs 8.0 cm in boys), while late in puberty, the increase in standing height is derived more from axial than appendicular growth (4.5 vs 1.5 cm in both sexes). Males have a 1- to 2-year longer prepubertal growth than females because puberty occurs later in males, resulting in greater sex differences in leg than trunk length (18).

During puberty, periosteal apposition increases bone width while endocortical resorption enlarges the medullary cavity (19). Net cortical thickness increases because periosteal apposition is greater than endocortical resorption. In girls, periosteal apposition decelerates earlier and medullary contracts in girls. The net effect of cessation of periosteal apposition and medullary contraction in girls is the construction of a bone with a smaller total cross-sectional size and medullary size but similar cortical thickness to boys. At the metaphyses of long bones, vBMD of the trabecular compartment remains constant from 5 years of age to young adulthood in both sexes. At this region, sex differences in BMC, vBMD and cross-sectional size emerges after puberty; males are reported to have thicker trabeculae and higher bone volume/total volume (BV/TV) (8).

As the size of the vertebral body increases during growth, the amount of bone within it increases so there is no increase in vBMD before puberty (9). At puberty, trabecular vBMD increases in both sexes and in African Americans and Caucasians, and is due to an increase in trabecular thickness rather than number. The increase is race-specific, but not different by sex (20). The vertebral body cross-section is ~15% larger in boys than girls before puberty and ~25% greater at maturity, but there is no sex difference in trabecular number or thickness. That is, the sex differences in morphology is in size, not apparent density; vertebral total cross-sectional area (CSA) but neither vertebral height nor trabecular density differ before puberty.

Incidence of fractures of the distal metaphysis of radius peaks at 10 to 12 years of age in girls and 12 to 14 years in boys, coinciding with the pubertal growth spurt (21). The rate of linear growth peaks earlier than that of bone mass. Growth of the radius is more rapid at the distal metaphysis and outpaces bone formation upon the surfaces of trabeculae emerging from the growth plate. Their coalescence forming the cortical bone of the metaphyseal region is delayed, producing a transient intracortical porosity predisposed to fracture (22,23). In late puberty, with slowing of longitudinal bone growth, trabeculae coalesce as bone formation proceeds on trabecular surfaces. Cortical porosity decreases and matrix mineralization increases, resulting in an increase in cortical vBMD. Exposure to sex steroids in peri- and postpubertal girls may enhance the consolidation of metaphyseal cortex at the endocortical surface, decreasing the residual cortical porosity earlier than in males (24,25).

The wider metaphysis must be modelled to fit the relatively slender diaphysis during longitudinal growth. Unlike the diaphysis where bone diameter increases by periosteal apposition, the metaphyseal cortex is resorbed from the periosteal surface while bone formation occurs upon the endocortical surface by trabecular coalescence. This resorptive modelling upon the periosteal surface and deposition of bone on the endocortical surface by corticalisation of trabeculae differs from diaphyseal cortical thickening by membranous bone formation.

The effects of illness during growth depend on the maturational stage at the time of disease exposure, not just the severity of the illness. As longitudinal growth is more rapid in the appendicular than axial skeleton before and in early puberty, illness may produce greater deficits in appendicular morphology. For example, disease affecting radial growth before puberty, and especially during early puberty, compromises the gain in bending strength. Illness during late puberty may produce greater deficits in the axial than the appendicular morphology, while in post-puberty is unlikely to produce deficits in bone size (26,27). This regional specificity in growth and the effects of illness are obscured by the study of standing height alone or BMD alone.

Diseases leading to sex hormone deficiency in females during puberty produce loss of sexual dimorphism in leg length, as estrogen deficiency allows continued growth in females so the epiphyses do not fuse and periosteal apposition continues. Periosteal apposition continues increasing bone width while endocortical apposition fails to occur, so cortical thickness is reduced, but only modestly, and the bone is wider. By contrast, the pubertal growth spurt in trunk length may be affected, creating a shorter but wider vertebral body and a shorter sitting height. Delayed puberty in males reduces periosteal apposition, producing a narrower bone with a thinner cortex, while appendicular growth in length continues producing a longer, more slender bone with a thinner cortex predisposing to greater fragility in males than females, as greater bone diameter in females with delayed puberty produces a biomechanical advantage and less cortical thinning because the lack of endocortical apposition is offset by continued periosteal apposition (28–30).

BONE LOSS DURING YOUNG ADULTHOOD

In young adulthood, bone remodelling maintains the material composition and structure of the skeleton by the focal resorption of a volume of old or damaged mineralized bone matrix from a surface by osteoclasts followed by formation of the same volume of new matrix at the same location by osteoblasts (31,32). This cellular level remodelling is undertaken by osteoclasts and osteoblasts, which constitute teams of short-lived cells forming the bone multicellular unit (BMU) (33).

Prior to menopause, the birth rate of new BMUs is slow and in steady state; the number of new BMUs excavating bone upon one or more of the three components of the endosteal surface equals the number of BMUs completing remodelling by bone formation. Although decreases in BMD are reported to occur before midlife, these data should be interpreted with caution (34,35). In the absence of a negative bone balance and slow bone remodelling, it is difficult to explain the reduction in bone density other than by a systematic measurement error produced perhaps by changes in marrow fat, which allows photon transmission producing a lower BMD interpreted as bone 'loss.' If there is bone loss prior menopause, the consequences are likely to be less than bone loss later in life because (i) remodelling rate is slow; (ii) trabecular bone loss probably proceeds by reduced bone formation rather than increased bone resorption by the BMU; (iii) bone loss proceeds by trabecular thinning rather than loss of connectivity so a given decrement in trabecular BMD produces less loss of strength than produced by loss of connectivity (36); and (iv) continued periosteal apposition partly offsets endocortical bone loss, thus shifting the cortices radially and maintaining cortical area and resistance to bending (37–39).

BONE LOSS DURING MENOPAUSE AND ADVANCING AGE

Advancing age is associated with four changes in the cellular machinery of bone modelling and remodelling that compromise bone's material properties and structural strength. There is a decline in the volume of bone formed by each BMU (40). This is the first age-related change in the cellular machinery. The second abnormality in remodelling is an increase in the volume of bone resorbed by the BMU, probably confined to a brief period following sex hormone deficiency (41). The opposite appears true during advancing age – the volume of bone resorbed by each BMU decreases, as reflected in a lower resorption cavity depth and an age-related increase, rather than decrease in interstitial thickness (interosteonal distance) (32,42,43). The third age-related abnormality is an increase in the rate of bone remodelling after menopause. This is accompanied by worsening of the negative bone balance in each BMU as the volume of bone resorbed increases and the volume of bone formed decreases in the many more BMUs now remodelling bone on the three (endocortical, intracortical and trabecular) components of its endosteal envelope (41,44).

The fourth abnormality is also a reduction in bone formation at the tissue level – bone modelling on the periosteal envelope slows precipitously after completion of longitudinal growth but continues slowly, so that bone diameters enlarge, but no more than a few millimeters during the next 60 years (37–39). This is insufficient to compensate for vigorous endosteal bone loss from the endocortical surface (producing cortical thinning), from the intracortical surface (producing intracortical porosity) and from the trabecular surface (producing trabecular thinning), thus complete loss of trabeculae and loss of connectivity.

Variance in the negative BMU balance is small compared with the variance in the rate of remodelling, so the rate of bone loss during menopause and ageing is driven more by differences in remodelling rate between individuals than differences in the size of the negative BMU balance between them (33). Thus, the rapidity of remodelling is an important determinant of bone loss, and the increase in remodelling rate in midlife and worsening of the negative BMU balance associated with estrogen deficiency are responsible for accelerated bone loss.

At menopause, steady state is perturbed by an increase in the birth rate of many new BMUs removing bone from the three components of the endosteal envelope while the fewer BMUs created before menopause only now complete remodelling by depositing bone (because the formation phase is delayed and proceeds slowly) (45). This perturbation produces the net acceleration in bone loss and a rapid decline in BMD. This acceleration in loss is the result of expansion of the transient deficit in bone matrix and mineral produced by this delay and slowness of refilling of the many excavated sites created after menopause (46,47).

This 'remodelling transient', or temporary deficit in bone mass and mineral, has three components: the excavation site that lacks osteoid and mineral, the osteoid that lacks mineral, and bone that has undergone primary but not secondary mineralization. Primary mineralisation occurs rapidly, whereas secondary mineralisation, the slow enlargement of crystals of calcium hydroxyapatite-like mineral, takes months to years to complete (48). At any time, there are osteons created in the immediate postmenopausal period and fewer, earlier created, osteons at various stages of completing secondary mineralization.

Bone loss slows in the 3 to 5 years following menopause, but not because remodelling rate slows. The rate of bone loss slows because steady state is restored at the new and higher remodelling rate. Now the large numbers of BMUs excavating resorption cavities are matched by completion of remodelling by bone formation the equally large numbers of BMUs created in early menopause. Bone loss continues at a faster rate than before menopause but at a slower rate than immediately after menopause because BMU balance is negative, perhaps more negative than before menopause, producing a permanent deficit in bone mass and mineral mass (45). The higher the remodelling rate and the more negative the BMU balance, the greater the bone loss and microstructural decay. If the worsening BMU balance produced by changes in the life span of osteoclasts and osteoblasts is temporary, and the negative BMU balance lessens but persists, the rate of loss will also lessen, but it will persist because bone loss is mainly driven by the high remodelling rate.

As remodelling is always initiated upon bone surfaces, and trabecular bone has more surface per unit bone volume than cortical bone, trabecular bone is remodelled faster than cortical bone – at least initially. Excavated resorption sites create stress 'concentrators' which predispose to micro-damage (as a small cut in a test tube makes it easy to snap) (49). The high remodelling rate and negative BMU balance produces trabecular thinning and complete loss of trabeculae. Increased resorption depth is more likely to produce perforation and complete loss of trabeculae than either greater numbers of resorption cavities or reduced formation in the BMU in women (50,51). The loss of trabeculae compromises bone strength more greatly than thinning.

As remodelling continues, trabeculae are lost and so their surfaces disappear but remodelling on endocortical surface continues, increasing the surface area (like folds of intestinal villae). Remodelling on the intracortical surface (haversian canals) increases intracortical porosity. Increased porosity due to increased numbers of pores and/or increased size of pores by coalescence of adjacent remodelling cavities increases the surface available for remodelling – 'trabecularizing' the cortex (52,53). Total bone surface either does not change (increasing in cortical bone, decreasing trabecular bone) or increases (in regions of cortical bone only) so that late in life, bone loss is more cortical than trabecular in origin. The continued remodelling at a similar intensity with its negative BMU balance, on the same amount or more surface, removes the same amount of bone from an ever-decreasing amount of bone, accelerating the loss of bone and structural decay.

Rapid remodelling also modifies the material properties of bone. More densely mineralised bone is removed and replaced with younger, less densely mineralized bone, reducing stiffness. Increased remodelling impairs isomerisation of collagen (54–58). Interstitial bone deep to surface remodelling becomes more densely mineralised and more highly cross-linked with advanced glycation end-products (AGEs) like pentosidine, both processes reducing bone toughness; it is easier for micro-cracks to lengthen through homogeneously mineralised bone.

Interstitial (interosteonal) bone has reduced osteocyte numbers and accumulates micro-damage (59).

Periosteal apposition is believed to increase as an adaptive response to compensate for the loss of strength produced by endocortical bone loss, so there will be no *net* loss of bone, no cortical thinning and no loss of bone strength. In a prospective study of over 600 women, Szulc et al. report that endocortical bone loss occurred in premenopausal women with concurrent periosteal apposition (39). As periosteal apposition was less than endocortical resorption, the cortices thinned but there was no *net* bone loss because the thinner cortex was now distributed around a larger perimeter conserving total bone mass. Moreover, resistance to bending increased despite bone loss and cortical thinning because this same amount of bone was now distributed further from the neutral axis (Figure 9.4).

During the perimenopausal period endocortical resorption increased, yet periosteal apposition decreased. The cortices thinned but bending strength remained unchanged despite bone loss and cortical thinning because periosteal apposition was still sufficient to shift the thinning cortex outwards. Bone fragility emerged only after menopause when accelerated in endocortical bone resorption and deceleration in periosteal apposition produce further cortical thinning.

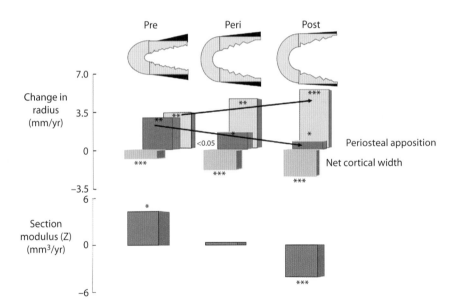

Figure 9.4 The amount of bone resorbed by endocortical resorption increases with age. The amount deposited by periosteal apposition decreases. The net effect is a decline in cortical thickness. In premenopausal women, the thinner cortex is displaced radially increasing section modulus (Z). In perimenopausal women, Z does not decrease despite cortical thinning because periosteal apposition still produces radial displacement. In postmenopausal women, Z decreases because endocortical resorption continues, periosteal apposition declines and little radial displacement occurs. (Adapted with permission from Szulc P et al. *J Bone Miner Res.* 2006;21(12):1856-63.)

As periosteal apposition was now minimal, there was little outward displacement of the thinning cortex, so cortical area now declined as did resistance to bending. During aging, both increasing endocortical bone resorption and reduced periosteal apposition cause *net* bone loss, alterations in the distribution of the remaining bone and the emergence of bone fragility.

SEX DIFFERENCES IN TRABECULAR AND CORTICAL BONE LOSS

A greater proportion of women than men sustain fragility fractures during their lifetime because men assemble a larger skeleton than women during growth so that resistance to bending is greater in men than women. Bone loss in men is the result of a negative BMU balance produced by reduced formation rather than increased resorption by the BMUs, so trabecular bone loss occurs by thinning rather than loss of connectivity (50). Men do not have a midlife decline in sex hormones and increase in remodelling rate that drives structural decay. Cortical porosity increases less in men than in women because remodelling rate is lower in men, and periosteal apposition may be greater in men than in women as reported in some studies (60,61).

SUMMARY AND CONCLUSION

Skeletal fragility in advanced age has its antecedence in growth because the variance in bone traits achieved during growth is an order of magnitude greater than rates of loss during aging. Factors modifying skeletal morphology such as exercise and nutrition are likely to be best during growth. Adaptive modelling by bone formation without resorption alters the size and shape of bone, while resorptive modelling during growth without bone formation excavates the marrow cavity. Bone remodelling, the resorption of a volume of bone followed by the deposition of a volume of bone at the same location by the cells of the BMU, is reparative but becomes unbalanced around midlife, compromising the integrity of the bone; a decline in the volume of bone formed by each BMU, continued resorption of a volume of bone by each BMU, an increase in remodelling rate in midlife in women and in both sexes late in life due to secondary hyperparathyroidism, and a decline in periosteal apposition result in the structural deterioration, because endosteal bone loss is not compensated by reduced periosteal bone formation.

A better understanding of the cellular mechanisms of bone modelling and remodelling and elucidation of the effects of advancing age on these mechanisms is likely to assist in identifying new targets for therapy that will help in preventing and reversing bone fragility. Advances in imaging allow quantification the material composition and microstructure of bone and so open doors to quantifying specific determinants of bone strength so that persons at risk for fracture can be identified and offered treatment.

REFERENCES

1. Seeman E. Growth in bone mass and size – Are racial and gender differences in bone mineral density more apparent than real? *J Clin Endocrinol Metab*. 1998;83(5):1414-9.
2. Hui SL, Slemenda CW, Johnston CC, Jr. The contribution of bone loss to postmenopausal osteoporosis. *Osteoporos Int*. 1990;1(1):30-4.
3. Bjornerem A, Johnsen SL, Nguyen TV, Kiserud T, Seeman E. The shifting trajectory of growth in femur length during gestation. *J Bone Miner Res*. 2010;25(5):1029-33.
4. Pietilainen KH, Kaprio J, Rasanen M, Winter T, Rissanen A, Rose RJ. Tracking of body size from birth to late adolescence: Contributions of birth length, birth weight, duration of gestation, parents' body size, and twinship. *Am J Epidemiol*. 2001;154(1):21-9.
5. Wang Q, Alen M, Nicholson P, Lyytikainen A, Suuriniemi M, Helkala E, et al. Growth patterns at distal radius and tibial shaft in pubertal girls: A 2-year longitudinal study. *J Bone Miner Res*. 2005;20(6):954-61.
6. Ruff C. Growth tracking of femoral and humeral strength from infancy through late adolescence. *Acta Paediatr*. 2005;94(8):1030-7.
7. Cheng S, Volgyi E, Tylavsky FA, Lyytikainen A, Tormakangas T, Xu L, et al. Trait-specific tracking and determinants of body composition: A 7-year follow-up study of pubertal growth in girls. *BMC Med*. 2009;7:5.
8. Loro ML, Sayre J, Roe TF, Goran MI, Kaufman FR, Gilsanz V. Early identification of children predisposed to low peak bone mass and osteoporosis later in life. *J Clin Endocrinol Metab*. 2000;85(10):3908-18.
9. Seeman E, Hopper JL, Bach LA, Cooper ME, Parkinson E, McKay J, et al. Reduced bone mass in daughters of women with osteoporosis. *N Engl J Med*. 1989;320(9):554-8.
10. Murray PD, Huxley JS. Self-differentiation in the grafted limb-bud of the chick. *J Anat*. Jul 1925;59(Pt 4):379-84.
11. Lanyon LE. Control of bone architecture by functional load bearing. *J Bone Miner Res*. 1992;7 Suppl 2:S369-75.
12. Wang Q, Cheng S, Alen M, Seeman E, Finnish Calex Study G. Bone's structural diversity in adult females is established before puberty. *J Clin Endocrinol Metab*. 2009;94(5):1555-61.
13. Zebaze RM, Jones A, Welsh F, Knackstedt M, Seeman E. Femoral neck shape and the spatial distribution of its mineral mass varies with its size: Clinical and biomechanical implications. *Bone*. 2005;37(2):243-52.
14. Ruff CB, Hayes WC. Subperiosteal expansion and cortical remodeling of the human femur and tibia with aging. *Science*. 1982;217(4563):945-8.
15. Bjornerem A, Bui QM, Ghasem-Zadeh A, Hopper JL, Zebaze R, Seeman E. Fracture risk and height: An association partly accounted for by cortical porosity of relatively thinner cortices. *J Bone Miner Res*. 2013;28(9):2017-26.

16. Boutroy S, Walker MD, Liu XS, McMahon DJ, Liu G, Guo XE, et al. Lower cortical porosity and higher tissue mineral density in Chinese American versus white women. *J Bone Miner Res.* 2014;29(3):551-61.

17. Karlberg J. The infancy-childhood growth spurt. *Acta Paediatr Scand Suppl.* 1990;367:111-8.

18. Tanner JM, Whitehouse RH. Clinical longitudinal standards for height, weight, height velocity, weight velocity, and stages of puberty. *Arch Disease Child.* Mar 1976;51(3):170-9.

19. Garn SM. The course of bone gain and the phases of bone loss. *Orthop Clin North Am.* Nov 1972;3(3):503-20.

20. Gilsanz V, Boechat MI, Roe TF, Loro ML, Sayre JW, Goodman WG. Gender differences in vertebral body sizes in children and adolescents. *Radiology.* 1994;190(3):673-7.

21. Cooper C, Dennison EM, Leufkens HG, Bishop N, van Staa TP. Epidemiology of childhood fractures in Britain: A study using the general practice research database. *J Bone Miner Res.* 2004;19(12):1976-81.

22. Cadet ER, Gafni RI, McCarthy EF, McCray DR, Bacher JD, Barnes KM, et al. Mechanisms responsible for longitudinal growth of the cortex: Coalescence of trabecular bone into cortical bone. *J Bone Joint Surg Am.* 2003;85-A(9):1739-48.

23. Wang Q, Wang XF, Iuliano-Burns S, Ghasem-Zadeh A, Zebaze R, Seeman E. Rapid growth produces transient cortical weakness: A risk factor for metaphyseal fractures during puberty. *J Bone Miner Res.* 2010;25(7):1521-6.

24. Wang Q, Nicholson PH, Suuriniemi M, Lyytikainen A, Helkala E, Alen M, et al. Relationship of sex hormones to bone geometric properties and mineral density in early pubertal girls. *J Clin Endocrinol Metab.* 2004;89(4):1698-703.

25. Rauch F, Schoenau E. Peripheral quantitative computed tomography of the distal radius in young subjects – New reference data and interpretation of results. *J Musculoskel Neuron Interact.* 2005;5(2):119-26.

26. Khosla S, Riggs BL, Atkinson EJ, Oberg AL, McDaniel LJ, Holets M, et al. Effects of sex and age on bone microstructure at the ultradistal radius: A population-based noninvasive in vivo assessment. *J Bone Miner Res.* 2006;21(1):124-31.

27. Seeman E, Karlsson MK, Duan Y. On exposure to anorexia nervosa, the temporal variation in axial and appendicular skeletal development predisposes to site-specific deficits in bone size and density: A cross-sectional study. *J Bone Miner Res.* 2000;15(11):2259-65.

28. Kirmani S, Christen D, van Lenthe GH, Fischer PR, Bouxsein ML, McCready LK, et al. Bone structure at the distal radius during adolescent growth. *J Bone Miner Res.* 2009;24(6):1033-42.

29. Havill LM, Mahaney MC, T LB, Specker BL. Effects of genes, sex, age, and activity on BMC, bone size, and areal and volumetric BMD. *J Bone Miner Res.* 2007;22(5):737-46.

30. Schoenau E, Neu CM, Rauch F, Manz F. Gender-specific pubertal changes in volumetric cortical bone mineral density at the proximal radius. *Bone*. 2002;31(1):110-3.

31. Hattner R, Epker BN, Frost HM. Suggested sequential mode of control of changes in cell behaviour in adult bone remodelling. *Nature*. 1965;206 (983):489-90.

32. Eriksen EF. Normal and pathological remodeling of human trabecular bone: Three dimensional reconstruction of the remodeling sequence in normals and in metabolic bone disease. *Endocr Rev*. 1986 Nov;7(4):379-408.

33. Parfitt A. Skeletal heterogeneity and the purposes of bone remodelling: Implications for the understanding of osteoporosis. In: Marcus R FD, Kelsey J, editors. *Osteoporosis*. San Diego, CA: Academic Press; 1996. p. 315-39.

34. Riggs BL, Melton LJ, Robb RA, Camp JJ, Atkinson EJ, McDaniel L, et al. A population-based assessment of rates of bone loss at multiple skeletal sites: Evidence for substantial trabecular bone loss in young adult women and men. *J Bone Miner Res*. 2008;23(2):205-14.

35. Riggs BL, Wahner HW, Melton LJ, 3rd, Richelson LS, Judd HL, Offord KP. Rates of bone loss in the appendicular and axial skeletons of women. Evidence of substantial vertebral bone loss before menopause. *J Clin Invest*. 1986;77(5):1487-91.

36. van der Linden JC, Homminga J, Verhaar JA, Weinans H. Mechanical consequences of bone loss in cancellous bone. *J Bone Miner Res*. 2001;16(3):457-65.

37. Balena R, Shih MS, Parfitt AM. Bone resorption and formation on the periosteal envelope of the ilium: A histomorphometric study in healthy women. *J Bone Miner Res*. 1992;7(12):1475-82.

38. Seeman E. Periosteal bone formation – A neglected determinant of bone strength. *N Engl J Med*. 2003;349(4):320-3.

39. Szulc P, Seeman E, Duboeuf F, Sornay-Rendu E, Delmas PD. Bone fragility: Failure of periosteal apposition to compensate for increased endocortical resorption in postmenopausal women. *J Bone Miner Res*. 2006;21(12):1856-63.

40. Lips P, Courpron P, Meunier PJ. Mean wall thickness of trabecular bone packets in the human iliac crest: Changes with age. *Calcif Tissue Res*. 1978;26(1):13-7.

41. Manolagas SC. Birth and death of bone cells: Basic regulatory mechanisms and implications for the pathogenesis and treatment of osteoporosis. *Endocr Rev*. 2000;21(2):115-37.

42. Vedi S, Compston JE, Webb A, Tighe JR. Histomorphometric analysis of bone biopsies from the iliac crest of normal British subjects. *Metabol Bone Dis Relat Res*. 1982;4(4):231-6.

43. Croucher PI, Garrahan NJ, Mellish RW, Compston JE. Age-related changes in resorption cavity characteristics in human trabecular bone. *Osteoporos Int*. 1991;1(4):257-61.

44. Eriksen EF, Langdahl B, Vesterby A, Rungby J, Kassem M. Hormone replacement therapy prevents osteoclastic hyperactivity: A histomorphometric study in early postmenopausal women. *J Bone Miner Res.* 1999;14(7):1217-21.

45. Seeman E, Martin TJ. Co-administration of antiresorptive and anabolic agents: A missed opportunity. *J Bone Miner Res.* 2015;30(5):753-64.

46. Parfitt AM. Morphological basis of bone mineral measurements: Transient and steady state effects of treatment in osteoporosis. *Miner Elecrolyte Metab.* 1980;4:273-87.

47. Parfitt AM. The cellular basis of bone remodeling: The quantum concept reexamined in light of recent advances in the cell biology of bone. *Calcif Tissue Int.* 1984;36 Suppl 1:S37-45.

48. Akkus O, Polyakova-Akkus A, Adar F, Schaffler MB. Aging of microstructural compartments in human compact bone. *J Bone Miner Res.* 2003;18(6):1012-9.

49. Hernandez CJ, Gupta A, Keaveny TM. A biomechanical analysis of the effects of resorption cavities on cancellous bone strength. *J Bone Miner Res.* 2006;21(8):1248-55.

50. Aaron JE, Makins NB, Sagreiya K. The microanatomy of trabecular bone loss in normal aging men and women. *Clin Orthop Relat Res.* 1987(215): 260-71.

51. Arlot ME, Delmas PD, Chappard D, Meunier PJ. Trabecular and endocortical bone remodeling in postmenopausal osteoporosis: Comparison with normal postmenopausal women. *Osteoporos Int.*1990;1(1):41-9.

52. Martin RB. Porosity and specific surface of bone. *Crit Rev Biomed Eng.* 1984;10(3):179-222.

53. Zebaze RM, Ghasem-Zadeh A, Bohte A, Iuliano-Burns S, Mirams M, Price RI, et al. Intracortical remodelling and porosity in the distal radius and post-mortem femurs of women: A cross-sectional study. *Lancet.* 2010;375(9727):1729-36.

54. Boivin G, Meunier PJ. Changes in bone remodeling rate influence the degree of mineralization of bone. *Connect Tissue Res.* 2002;43(2-3):535-7.

55. Viguet-Carrin S, Garnero P, Delmas PD. The role of collagen in bone strength. *Osteoporos Int.* 2006;17(3):319-36.

56. Bailey AJ, Sims TJ, Ebbesen EN, Mansell JP, Thomsen JS, Mosekilde L. Age-related changes in the biochemical properties of human cancellous bone collagen: Relationship to bone strength. *Calcif Tissue Int.* 1999;65(3):203-10.

57. Banse X, Sims TJ, Bailey AJ. Mechanical properties of adult vertebral cancellous bone: Correlation with collagen intermolecular cross-links. *J Bone Miner Res.* 2002;17(9):1621-8.

58. Boivin G, Lips P, Ott SM, Harper KD, Sarkar S, Pinette KV, et al. Contribution of raloxifene and calcium and vitamin D3 supplementation to the increase of the degree of mineralization of bone in postmenopausal women. *J Clin Endocrinol Metab,* 2003;88(9):4199-205.

59. Seeman E, Delmas PD. Bone quality – The material and structural basis of bone strength and fragility. *N Engl J Med.* 2006;354(21):2250-61.

60. Duan Y, Beck TJ, Wang XF, Seeman E. Structural and biomechanical basis of sexual dimorphism in femoral neck fragility has its origins in growth and aging. *J Bone Miner Res.* 2003;18(10):1766-74.

61. Duan Y, Turner CH, Kim BT, Seeman E. Sexual dimorphism in vertebral fragility is more the result of gender differences in age-related bone gain than bone loss. *J Bone Miner Res.* 2001;16(12):2267-75.

Risk factors for post peak bone loss and osteoporotic fracture: Lessons from population studies

BO ABRAHAMSEN

INTRODUCTION

Osteoporotic fractures arise from compromised strength of the skeleton. The ability for bones to withstand trauma without fracturing can be predicted in part by their content of calcium. This is most often assessed by dual-energy X-ray absorptiometry (DXA), which is the current gold standard, though other techniques exist and pose some advantages (1). As one cannot easily determine skeletal strength, clinicians and epidemiologists have to rely on indirect evidence that a fracture is due to osteoporosis. While low energy fractures can be identified in cohort studies on fracture risk by carefully inquiring into the circumstances leading up to the fracture, fracture epidemiology generally relies on some fractures being more likely to be secondary to osteoporosis than others. For fractures of the hip, spine, humerus and forearm, the relationship with low bone mineral density (BMD) and advancing age is strong enough for these fracture locations to be treated epidemiologically as major osteoporotic fractures. It is well established that patients with osteoporosis are also at increased risk of fractures at other locations, and that includes fractures arising after high energy trauma (2). This chapter addresses risk factors for osteoporotic fractures and bone loss in adults after the time at which peak bone mass is attained. Other chapters address determinants of peak bone mass.

We can group risk factors for fracture in several ways: modifiable or non-modifiable, acquired or innate, strong or weak, common or rare, important in both sexes or in one, linked to many fracture sites or few. Clearly, initiatives to improve public health must aim at successfully addressing strong, prevalent, modifiable risk factors. Such risk factors include alcohol and tobacco habits, frailty and a range of medication exposures, but conclusive intervention studies are generally lacking (3). Non-modifiable risk factors such as a family history of osteoporosis or a history of prior fractures nevertheless are important to clinical management as they may allow targeting of resources towards persons who are at increased risk of sustaining future osteoporotic fractures (4). Even the rarest genetic causes of osteoporosis may identify new pathophysiological mechanisms that can be used to develop therapeutics that can be helpful in the management of osteoporosis in a broad population: osteoprotegerin, sclerostin and cathepsin K are all examples of this (5,6).

There are some deliberate omissions in this chapter. First, the FRAX® algorithm is the subject of Chapter 12 and is not addressed here. Second, a large number of common gene variants, each with moderate or small influence on adult bone health, have been identified and are addressed in Chapter 1.

In the following, factors influencing rates of bone loss are described based on the relatively small number of population-based cohort studies with sequential BMD measurements. By contrast, fractures can be captured not only in face-to-face prospective cohort studies but also in national health registries, claims databases and general practice records. Such studies permit a lower level of phenotypic detail but may offer a higher degree of external validity over studies that actively recruit volunteers.

Observational studies in the fracture area have used a case-control design, or more commonly, a cohort design. A useful review of the advantages and disadvantages of these two distinct approaches is provided elsewhere (7). The key difference is that case-control studies compare groups of subjects who do or do not develop a given outcome, while cohort studies compare groups of subjects who do or do not have a certain exposure. The main advantages of the cohort study are that absolute event rates can be calculated and that more than one outcome can be pursued.

RISK FACTORS FOR BONE LOSS

For this review it was possible to identify a very modest number of cohort studies (Table 10.1) addressing risk factor status specifically in relation to adult bone loss rates, with most studies reporting on a small number of risk factors with significant associations with bone loss rates. The precision of rate-of-changes

Table 10.1 Observational cohort studies on adult bone loss rates

Study	Modifiable risk factors	Non-modifiable risk factors
CaMos	Low calcium and vitamin D intake (16)	
Rotterdam	Low BMI, smoking, low calcium intake in men (8)	
Dubbo Osteoporosis Epidemiology Study (DOES)	Low FM in women but not in men (9)	
SOF	Higher BTMs (30) Low vitamin D and sex hormones (17) Low vegetable protein intake (31) Low B12 (28) Weight loss (10)	Type 2 diabetes (25)
MrOS	Low 25(OH)D (18) Peripheral artery disease (32)	
Tobago Health Study (M)	GFR < 60 (27)	
EPIC Norfolk	Weight loss, low physical activity, low vitamin C intake (11)	
Health ABC study	Low HCO3 levels (33)	Diabetes, but sex/ ethnicity specific (26)
Hertfordshire study	BMI and BMI change (12)	
HUNT	Midlife weight loss (13)	
Kuopio OSTPRE	No effect of obesity (15) or statins (34)	
Michigan Bone Health and Metabolism Study	Menopausal transition, FSH level stage (19) Age 20–54: Low alcohol intake, lack of sports participation	Increased loss: Reproductive cancer (20)
Muramatsu cohort	Overall nutritional status, weight loss (35)	
SWAN	BMI (14)	Ethnicity (14)
Tromsø Study	Weak correlation with sex steroids and SHBG (21)	

Note: BTM: bone turnover markers; FM: fat mass; FSH: follicle stimulating hormone; GFR: glomerular filtration rate; M: males; SHBG: sex hormone binding globulin.

estimates is inherently poorer than that of a single BMD measurement, and it stands to reason that otherwise well-powered cohorts may encounter difficulties in reliably differentiating between the relative importance of risk factors which may also show interaction or collinearity. In general, low body mass index (BMI) and weight loss were found to be linked with higher bone loss rates, while higher BMI, fat mass and weight gain had the opposite effect in the majority (8–14), but not all (15), studies. Both higher vitamin D and higher calcium intake had a favourable association with longitudinal change in BMD in adult Canadian women, with inconclusive effects in men (16) in the the Canadian Multicentre Osteoporosis Study (CaMos). In both women and men, however, higher serum levels of vitamin D were associated with lower bone loss rates as assessed in the Study of Osteoporotic Fractures (17), and in MrOs (18). In women, lower sex hormone levels, menopausal transition and a history of reproductive cancer have all been found to be predictive of accelerated bone loss rates in observational cohorts (17,19–21), in line with the physiological actions of female sex hormones on the activation frequency within trabecular and cortical bone (22–24). Comorbid conditions such as type 2 diabetes (25,26), mildly reduced renal function (27) and vitamin B12 deficiency (28) all appear to be associated with increased adult bone loss rates, though the information is based on a small number of cohorts. In a modestly sized study of BMD changes at menopause in 862 US women, the slowest bone loss rates were observed in African American women and the fastest in women of Japanese or Chinese ethnicity, indicating racial differences in postmenopausal bone loss rates (14). The genes involved in regulation of bone loss rates are addressed in a separate chapter and are not reviewed here, but it is useful to be mindful of the relatively low apparent heritability of bone loss rates – as opposed to BMD itself – in twins, and the gradual decline in heritability of loss rates with age (29). This suggests that, at least in the older age segment, risk factors for bone loss are largely acquired rather than inherited, hence leaving public health strategies with several points of potential intervention perhaps particularly targeted to persons at risk of malnutrition or who suffer from poorly controlled chronic comorbid conditions that are treatable.

MODIFIABLE RISK FACTORS FOR FRACTURE (TABLE 10.2)

Lifestyle

Alcohol and tobacco are two strong, modifiable lifestyle factors. Thus, smoking has consistently been associated with an increased risk of spine (36) and hip fractures, as addressed originally in a 2005 meta-analysis (37). One of the most extensively studied cohorts in this context is the MrOS study, where the latest analysis in the US subcohort, with 5994 men aged 65+ and a mean follow-up of almost 9 years, demonstrated a threefold increased hip fracture risk in men who were current smokers (38). Interestingly, the association remained strong and pronounced (HR 2.05; 95% CI 1.05-3.98) even after adjusting for femoral neck BMD, demonstrating that the risk is not fully captured by BMD alone. Vertebral fracture has also been linked to current smoking; in the Study of Osteoporotic

Table 10.2 Modifiable and non-modifiable risk factors for fracture

Study	FRAX development cohort	FRAX validation cohort	Modifiable risk factors	Non-modifiable risk factors
CaMos	x		Low protein intake (131), 'a frailty index' (51), GC use (132), low QoL (133)	
Cardiovascular Health Study			Albuminuria: Increased risk of hip fracture (modest) in women but not in men (134) Heart failure: Increased risk of hip fracture (135) Alcohol consumption, U-shaped relationship with hip fracture (42)	High levels of soluble CD14 marks increased risk (136) Low levels of circulating TGF beta1 associated with higher hip fracture risk in women with variable to decreased risk in men (137)
DOPS			Beta blocker users had higher fracture risk (138); NSAID users higher risk (139) High PTH levels combined with low vitamin D increased risk (77)	
Dubbo Osteoporosis Epidemiology Study (DOES)	x		Increased risk with OA (140) and hypertension (141) Beta-blockers (142,143) protective Lower serum testosterone = higher fracture risk in 60+ men (62)	

(Continued)

Table 10.2 (Continued) Modifiable and non-modifiable risk factors for fracture

Study	FRAX development cohort	FRAX validation cohort	Modifiable risk factors	Non-modifiable risk factors
EPIC Norfolk			*Magnesium intake protective but not when adjusted for multiple testing (144)*	
EVOS/EPOS	×		Amenorrhea (36,96), falls (56), body weight (36,92), alcohol, smoking (36)	Late menarche (36,96), family hip fracture (96), prior vertebral fracture (91), prior hip fracture (92)
Framingham heart study				Recent height loss in elderly men and women predicted risk of hip fracture (145)
Framingham osteoporosis study			Vitamin C supplements (unlike dietary) – lower risk of hip fracture (146) Higher HCy levels (147) and coffee consumption increased hip fracture risk (148)	
Geelong		×	Depression (149) Lower fracture risk in beta-blocker users (150) Urban population higher fracture risk (151)	

(Continued)

Table 10.2 (Continued) Modifiable and non-modifiable risk factors for fracture

Study	FRAX development cohort	FRAX validation cohort	Modifiable risk factors	Non-modifiable risk factors
GLOW			Hip fracture predictors: Weight, falls, weight loss, lack of physical activity Spine fracture predictors: Weight, weight loss, asthma, physical inactivity (47,46) Body weight protective for major osteoporotic fracture while opposite effect on ankle fractures (44)	Hip fracture predictors: Age, prior fracture Spine fracture predictors: Age, prior fracture, poor health (47)
Kuopio OSTPRE			Physical function and postmenopausal fractures (152) Higher body mass index decreased the risk of wrist fracture while increasing that of ankle fracture (153)	
Million Women			BMI and physical activity influence fracture risk in postmenopausal women but direction of effect depends on anatomical site (48)	Increased risk in taller women (154)
MONICA Augsburg			Beta-blocker users had lower fracture risk (155)	

(Continued)

Table 10.2 (Continued) Modifiable and non-modifiable risk factors for fracture

Study	FRAX development cohort	FRAX validation cohort	Modifiable risk factors	Non-modifiable risk factors
MrOS			Low 25(OH)D (18)	Inflammatory cytokines increased risk (164)
			Smoking, use of tricyclic antidepressants (70), lower protein intake and lower executive function (38)	Higher hip fracture risk: Greater height and height loss since age 25, history of fracture, history of myocardial infarction or angina, hyperthyroidism or Parkinson disease (70)
			Increased risk if hyponatremia (156)	Type, number and location of prior vertebral fractures in men influence risk of subsequent fractures (93)
			Increased risk with low cobalamins (157)	
			Increased fracture risk if low serum E2 and high SHBG levels (63) or low free testosterone (64)	Increased risk of vertebral fractures if high SHBG (69)
			Also combination of low bioavailable testosterone and low vitamin D status increased risk (158)	Increased risk: High U-Cadmium excretion (165)
			Body composition (159)	Increased risk if accelerated bone loss (166)
			Sarcopenia (160)	Serum adiponectin and short-term risk (167)
			Subclinical hyperthyreosis increased risk hip fracture (161)	Higher risk of nonspine fractures with low uric acid levels (128)
			Obesity, adjusted for BMD, increased risk (162)	
			Recurrent falls (163)	

(Continued)

Table 10.2 (Continued) Modifiable and non-modifiable risk factors for fracture

Study	FRAX development cohort	FRAX validation cohort	Modifiable risk factors	Non-modifiable risk factors
			Frailty (52) and poor physical function (53)	Aortic calcification – increased hip fracture risk (168) Renal function but may not be independent predictor, also method dependent (108) Higher FGF-23 – increased risk of fractures (169)
Nagano Cohort study			Low vitamin D levels increase risk of hip and other long bone fractures (170)	
NHANES III				Hb-levels biphasic association, increased risk if high or low levels (171)
NOREPOS			Increased if low vitamin K1 (172)	
Nurses' Health Study			Diuretics and vertebral fractures (173) Increased risk of hip fracture in low physical activity women with abdominal obesity controlled for BMI (49) Increased risk if nightshift work (174)	Plasma oxidative stress markers an independent risk factor for fracture (177)

(Continued)

Table 10.2 (Continued) Modifiable and non-modifiable risk factors for fracture

Study	FRAX development cohort	FRAX validation cohort	Modifiable risk factors	Non-modifiable risk factors
			Western dairy pattern not a risk factor for fracture (175)	
			Increased soda consumption increased hip fracture risk (176)	
			Smoking (40)	
OFELY			HCy levels but not if adjusted for age (178)	Vertebral shape (179)
				High serum periostin increased risk (180)
OPUS		×	Low estradiol increased fracture risk (66)	
OPRA, Malmoe			Smoking (41)	
			balance, gait speed and self-reported history of fall (57)	
Rochester cohorts	×		Pernicious anaemia (181), PHPT (182), AS (183)	
Rotterdam	×		A-vitamin (184), hyponatremia (185), B-vitamins (186), T4 (187), HCy (188)	Uric acid (127), lumbar disc degeneration (189), SHBG (190)

(Continued)

Table 10.2 (Continued) Modifiable and non-modifiable risk factors for fracture

Study	FRAX development cohort	FRAX validation cohort	Modifiable risk factors	Non-modifiable risk factors
Singapore Chinese Health Study			Lower risk with higher free estradiol and E2 bioactivity (67) Vegetable consumption and carotenoids inversely related with hip fracture risk (191) Tofu, soy and isoflavone intake protective (hip), though not in men (192)	
SOF		×	Decline in lower extremity physical performance (54) BVF loss increased fracture risk (193) Lower prevalence of vertebral fractures if higher estradiol level (68)	Surgical menopause no increased fracture risk (143)
Swedish Mammography cohort			Low alpha-tocopherol (194) Below five servings of fruit and vegetables associated with increased risk of hip fracture (195) Minor importance vitamin D intake (196)	

(Continued)

Table 10.2 (Continued) Modifiable and non-modifiable risk factors for fracture

Study	FRAX development cohort	FRAX validation cohort	Modifiable risk factors	Non-modifiable risk factors
Tromsø Study			Physical activity is associated with reduced fracture risk at weight-bearing sites, with no associations at non-weight-bearing sites (50)	Height (199)
			Increased non-vertebral fracture risk in diabetic women who smoke (197)	
			Self-reported comorbidities (198)	
Uppsala ULSAM			Low alpha-tocopherol (194)	
WHI		x	Lower risk in women with preference for wine over other drinks or compared with non-drinkers (43)	Nephrolithiasis – increased risk but not after adjustments (203)
			Anaemia higher risk of fractures (200)	Non-surgical menopause <40y of age (121)
			Saturated fat intake, higher risk (201)	Moderate or severe menopausal vasomotor symptoms associated with increased hip fracture risk (204)
			Depressive symptoms and spine fractures (202)	High OPG levels predict increased hip fracture risk (205)
			Higher vitamin D levels protective but only in white women (76)	Renal function as assessed by cystatin C levels but some differed by ethnicity (109)

Note: Italics denote negative findings. BVF, binocular visual field; GC, glucocorticoid; HCy, homocysteine; NSAID, non-steroid anti-inflammatory drugs; OA, osteoarthrosis; PHPT, primary hyperparathyroidism; PTH, parathyroid hormone; QoL, quality of life; SHBG, sex hormone binding globulin; TGF, transforming growth factor.

Fractures, current smokers were at 1.7 times the risk of radiographic vertebral fractures compared with non-smokers (39). Smoking is clearly a modifiable risk factor and there is evidence both from the Nurses' Health Study (40) and more recently the Swedish OPRA study (41) that the risk of osteoporotic fractures declines after smoking cessation in women. The former study reported a 30% lower hip fracture risk ten years after participants had stopped smoking, while the latter study, which was smaller and had a shorter follow-up time, found a decrease of 11% in overall fracture risk with each year after cessation, albeit driven without any appreciable effect on hip fracture risk. The fracture risks associated with excessive alcohol consumption are undisputed but there is some doubt as to the safe level. Unfortunately, the definition of a unit of alcohol varies across countries and this has led to some confusion in the past. Moreover, a zero consumption of alcohol at present may indicate either a lifelong history of complete abstinence or its opposite, a history of alcohol abuse. By contrast, a small consumption of alcohol is more likely a sign of a lifetime of moderation. This paradox can bias epidemiological analyses in the direction of one unit of alcohol daily reducing the risk of adverse outcomes. A U-shaped relationship between alcohol intake and fractures has been apparent in several studies. In the Cardiovascular Health study of US subjects above 65 years of age, participants who consumed up to 14 drinks per week were at about 20% lower risk of hip fracture than long-term abstainers, while the risk was about 20% higher among consumers of 14 or more drinks per week (42). For vertebral fractures, alcohol consumption 5 days a week or over was associated with no significant increase in risk in either sex, though the effect estimate was within the confidence range of that reported from the Cardiovascular Health Study for the hip (36). In men in the United States followed in the MrOs cohort, researchers found a nominal lower risk of hip fractures in men with an intake of more than 14 units a week, though this was not statistically significant when corrected for BMD (38). A preference for wine over other drinks was associated with lower fracture risk in women (43) in the Women's Health Initiative.

Obesity is a modifiable risk factor for some fractures, but the relationship is complex (44,45). Obesity has been found to offer some protection against major osteoporotic fractures, while a risk factor for other fractures – in particular those of the lower leg and ankle. In the primary practice cohort-based GLOW study, the associations with weight and BMI differed substantially across anatomical sites, with BMI being strongly negatively correlated with hip, spine and wrist fractures, while increasing body weight increased the risk of ankle fractures (44). Upper arm and clavicle fractures were associated with height rather than weight. Further, unintentional weight loss increased the risk of hip and other fractures for up to 5 years in this cohort (46).

Low physical activity, disability and falls may or may not be modifiable, depending on the condition. Low physical activity (47–50), frailty (51,52) and disability (38,53–55) have all been associated with increased risk of fractures in observational cohorts, as have falls (47,56,57). Unsurprisingly, fall risk-increasing drugs such as opioids, dopaminergics, antidepressants and sedatives all increase the risk of hip fracture (58), and sleep disturbances in themselves increase the risk of falls (59). A significant reduction in the risk of falling can be achieved through multidisciplinary intervention including training programmes and home safety interventions (60). Observations in the Study of Osteoporotic Fractures suggested that the type of fall resulting in a hip fracture differs from the type of fall that leads to wrist fractures (61).

Endocrine factors

Endocrine predictors of fracture risk include male (62–65) and female (66–68) gonadal hormone levels, sex hormone–binding globulin (69) have also been shown to correlate with fracture risk to a variable degree in population studies. Discrepancies between studies may be partly attributable to differences in the performance of the assays used, which can be challenging due to the relatively low levels of bioavailable sex steroids in older men and in postmenopausal women. Hyperthyroidism is another potentially modifiable condition that has been linked to fracture risk in most but not all population studies. In the MrOs study, a history of hyperthyroidism was one of the comorbid conditions linked to risk of hip fractures (70), while the Cardiovascular Health Study found no such association (71) in a cohort of 4936 US adults. One major difficulty is accounting in full for changes in thyroid status over time, and the introduction of thyroid medications post-baseline. Linkage of Danish healthcare databases to biochemistry information found that the risk of fractures increased in patients with hyperthyroidism and particularly those with long-standing subclinical disease (72), a finding that is in line with a recent meta-analysis covering 13 large prospective cohorts (73). Where thyroid disorders are a broad spectrum of disorders ranging from self-limiting acute or subacute disease to chronic states of thyroid hormone deficiency or excess, diabetes should principally be regarded as a cluster of chronic, though in some cases eminently treatable, diseases. Because of this, diabetes will be dealt with under non-modifiable risk factors below.

Nutrition and fracture risk

Vitamin D is essential for active calcium absorption in the gut, for normal skeletal mineralisation and for maintaining normocalcaemia and normal muscle function. The desirable serum level of vitamin D has been the subject of some controversy (74) but suffice it to say that there is little evidence that fracture risk is higher in subjects with serum levels of 50 nmol/L, the levels recommended by the US Institute of Medicine, than in those with 75 nmol/L, a level often supported, particularly in the US. Several observational cohorts (Table 10.2) have reported on the risk of fractures in subjects with low vitamin D levels but results have been variable, though with a more consistent relationship in newer cohorts, likely attributable to advances in vitamin D assays. For a comprehensive review of the controversies and knowledge gaps regarding vitamin D, vitamin D measurements and appropriate levels in different ethnic groups, readers are referred to the excellent paper by Fuleihan (75). Among recent, large population cohorts, both the MrOs study (18) and the WHI study (76) found inverse associations between vitamin D levels and the risk of fractures, though the latter study noted that the associations differed widely by ethnic group, with risk reductions with higher vitamin D levels confined to white women alone. In Danish postmenopausal women, low vitamin D levels were predictive of fractures only in the presence of elevated parathyroid hormone (PTH) (77).

Fracture and drug exposures

Medications may in themselves increase impact on skeletal strength as in the case for glucocorticoids and aromatase inhibitors, they may increase the risk of falling as in the case of hypnotics and anxiolytics, or they may be no more than an indicator of a comorbid condition which is associated with fracture risk (78). For example, if the entire portfolio of medications used in a population of patients with fractures is compared to that of age-matched non-fracture controls, medications such as iron, B12 and folate supplements associate with fracture risk as do more obvious candidates such as glucocorticoids, antidepressants and opioids (79). This does not necessarily imply that stopping iron supplements will cut fracture risk, but only that patients requiring such supplements could be a group of patients deserving of our attention in terms of osteoporosis diagnosis, treatment or prevention of falls. The presence of a dose-response relationship, recent rather than past exposure, a biologically plausible mechanism and evidence from animal models are some of the Bradford-Hill criteria that can help us make some inferences about which associations are causal (and perhaps modifiable) and which associations provide an opportunity for case finding. Much of what has been done on associations between fractures and drug exposures comes from prescription databases linked to administrative outcomes data rather than from physical clinic based cohorts. Critically, however, the latter studies are sometimes able to provide BMD information and functional tests to illuminate the mechanisms. A review of all drugs that are associated, at least in some but not necessarily all analyses, with an increased risk of fractures is beyond the scope of this chapter but such a list includes glucocorticoids (80,81), anti-androgens (82,83), aromatase inhibitors (84), excessive doses of thyroxine (85) and proton-pump inhibitors (86–88). Fracture risk is also modestly increased with anti-epileptics (89,90).

NON-MODIFIABLE ATTRIBUTES AND COMORBIDITIES AS RISK FACTORS FOR FRACTURE (TABLE 10.2)

The most prevalent, strong, non-modifiable risk factors for fractures in late adulthood are prior fractures (47,91–93) and age (47,94,95). A family history of osteoporotic fractures is also a prevalent and important risk factor for major osteoporotic fractures in the adult population (95–97). Regarding the specific genes contributing to adult fracture risk, please refer to Chapter 1 in this book. The relationship between bone geometry and structure and risk of fractures is also addressed elsewhere (Chapters 3 and 9) and is not covered in the present chapter. The degree of reversibility of chronic diseases that affect the risk of fractures varies, and so do the effects on bone. The effects of thyrotoxicosis (98–102) on the skeleton are reversible, at least in the short term, as are the physiological skeletal effects that take place during pregnancy and lactation. Even glucocorticoid excess – be it iatrogenic or endogenous – shows a remarkably short recovery time in the average patient, though severe vertebral fractures may occur with surprisingly short treatment courses and only moderate cumulative doses (80,81).

As reviewed in detail elsewhere (103), both type 1 and type 2 diabetes are associated with considerably increased risk of fracture in the individual patient, though the relative impact on total societal fracture burden is relatively modest (population attributable risk 4–10%). Paradoxically, patients with diabetes appear to be less likely to receive osteoporosis treatment despite their elevated fracture risk (104), possibly due to the relatively conserved BMD seen in type 2 diabetes with an altered fracture threshold (more fractures at the same BMD level), and also likely influenced by the higher prevalence of reduced renal function in diabetes populations, which can preclude the use of anti-fracture medications. As fracture incidence appears to be higher in patients with complications to diabetes (105) – potentially partly due to the increased risk of falls but also likely due to collagen modifications and other changes to the composition of bone (106) – it is reasonable to assume that improved diabetes control will also reduce the risk of fractures.

The list of chronic diseases that should be considered risk factors for adult fractures is long and includes impaired renal function (107–109), organ transplantation (110,111), primary hyperparathyroidism (112), inflammatory bowel diseases (hip fracture [113,114], vertebral fracture [115]), coeliac disease (116,117), anorexia (118–120), late menarche (36,96), amenorrhea (36,96), early menopause (121), rheumatoid arthritis (122,123) and ankylosing spondylitis. Gout (124–126) and uric acid levels (127) may or may not be risk factors for osteoporotic fracture. However, serum uric acid levels themselves have shown a negative correlation with fracture risk in some cohorts (128), and the evidence on the effects of allopurinol on bone also remains somewhat conflicting. With substantial improvements in cancer treatment, a growing number of cancer survivors (129) become subject to bone fragility as a consequence of anti-hormonal therapy, chemotherapy, radiation therapy and/or glucocorticoid treatment. Another area of concern in terms of bone health is bariatric surgery, where effects on bone mass and fracture risk (130) are becoming increasingly apparent and recognised.

CONCLUSIONS

While much information has been collected from population-based cohort studies to help us understand risk factors for fracture, our understanding of determinants of bone loss rates at population level is still relatively limited, with menopause, glucocorticoid excess, weight loss, compromised renal function and diabetes being the key areas investigated. After more than 25 years of DXA it is disappointing that so relatively little has been published on risk factors for accelerated bone loss; studies comparing and contrasting various risk factors within the same longitudinal BMD population would be particularly valuable for an understanding of their relative contribution and the interaction between them. Our understanding of risk factors for fracture in population-based studies, many of them eminently modifiable, is substantial and growing. However, it is clear from Table 10.2 that the overlap between what was studied in different cohorts is quite small, and it is difficult to know if other risk factors may have been the subject of negative studies that could perhaps not be published. For fracture risk factors, too it would be of particular value to collate multiple risk factors into comprehensive analyses to identify areas where intervention studies would have the greatest chance of success and areas where strong non-modifiable risk factors could be selected for targeted fracture prevention.

REFERENCES

1. Høiberg MP, Rubin KH, Hermann AP, Brixen K, Abrahamsen B. Diagnostic devices for osteoporosis in the general population: A systematic review. *Bone.* 2016;92:58-69.
2. Mackey DC et al. High-trauma fractures and low bone mineral density in older women and men. *JAMA.* 2007;298:2381-8.
3. Abrahamsen B, Brask-Lindemann D, Rubin KH, Schwarz P. A review of lifestyle, smoking and other modifiable risk factors for osteoporotic fractures. *Bonekey Rep.* 2014;3:574.
4. Leslie WD, Schousboe JT. A review of osteoporosis diagnosis and treatment options in new and recently updated guidelines on case finding around the world. *Curr Osteoporos Rep.* 2011;9:129-40.
5. Boudin E, Fijalkowski I, Hendrickx G, Van Hul W. Genetic control of bone mass. *Mol Cell Endocrinol.* 2016;432:3-13.
6. Schwarz P, Jørgensen NR, Abrahamsen B. Status of drug development for the prevention and treatment of osteoporosis. *Expert Opin Drug Discov.* 2014;9:245-53.
7. Vandenbroucke JP, et al. Strengthening the Reporting of Observational Studies in Epidemiology (STROBE): Explanation and elaboration. *Epidemiology.* 2007;18:805-35.
8. Burger H, et al. Risk factors for increased bone loss in an elderly population: The Rotterdam Study. *Am J Epidemiol.* 1998;147:871-9.
9. Yang S, Center JR, Eisman JA, Nguyen TV. Association between fat mass, lean mass, and bone loss: The Dubbo osteoporosis epidemiology study. *Osteoporos Int.* 2015;26:1381-6.
10. Ensrud KE, et al. Intentional and unintentional weight loss increase bone loss and hip fracture risk in older women. *J Am Geriatr Soc.* 2003; 51:1740-7.
11. Kaptoge S, et al. Effects of dietary nutrients and food groups on bone loss from the proximal femur in men and women in the 7th and 8th decades of age. *Osteoporos Int.* 2003;14:418-28.
12. Dennison E, et al. Determinants of bone loss in elderly men and women: A prospective population-based study. *Osteoporos Int.* 1999;10:384-91.
13. Forsmo S, Langhammer A, Schei B. Past and current weight change and forearm bone loss in middle-aged women: The Nord-Trøndelag Health Study, Norway. *Menopause.* 2009;16:1197-1204.

14. Greendale GA, et al. Bone mineral density loss in relation to the final menstrual period in a multiethnic cohort: Results from the Study of Women's Health Across the Nation (SWAN). *J Bone Miner Res.* 2012;27:111-8.

15. Saarelainen J, et al. Body mass index and bone loss among postmenopausal women: The 10-year follow-up of the OSTPRE cohort. *J Bone Miner Metab.* 2012;30:208-16.

16. Zhou W, et al. Longitudinal changes in calcium and vitamin D intakes and relationship to bone mineral density in a prospective population-based study: The Canadian Multicentre Osteoporosis Study (CaMos). *J Musculoskelet Neuronal Interact.* 2013;13:470-9.

17. Stone K, et al. Hormonal predictors of bone loss in elderly women: A prospective study. The Study of Osteoporotic Fractures Research Group. *J Bone Miner Res.* 1998;13:1167-74.

18. Swanson CM, et al. Associations of 25-hydroxyvitamin D and 1,25-dihydroxyvitamin D with bone mineral density, bone mineral density change, and incident nonvertebral fracture. *J Bone Miner Res.* 2015;30:1403-13.

19. Sowers MR, et al. Amount of bone loss in relation to time around the final menstrual period and follicle-stimulating hormone staging of the transmenopause. *J Clin Endocrinol Metab.* 2010;95:2155-62.

20. Bainbridge KE, Sowers M, Lin X, Harlow SD. Risk factors for low bone mineral density and the 6-year rate of bone loss among premenopausal and perimenopausal women. *Osteoporos Int.* 2004;15:439-46.

21. Bjørnerem A, et al. Circulating sex steroids, sex hormone-binding globulin, and longitudinal changes in forearm bone mineral density in postmenopausal women and men: The Tromsø Study. *Calcif Tissue Int.* 2007;81:65-72.

22. Brockstedt H, Kassem M, Eriksen EF, Mosekilde L, Melsen F. Age- and sex-related changes in iliac cortical bone mass and remodeling. *Bone.* 1993;14:681-91.

23. Parfitt AM, et al. Effects of ethnicity and age or menopause on osteoblast function, bone mineralization, and osteoid accumulation in iliac bone. *J Bone Miner Res.* 1997;12:1864-73.

24. Recker R, Lappe J, Davies KM, Heaney R. Bone remodeling increases substantially in the years after menopause and remains increased in older osteoporosis patients. *J Bone Miner Res.* 2004;19:1628-33.

25. Schwartz AV, et al. Diabetes and change in bone mineral density at the hip, calcaneus, spine, and radius in older women. *Front Endocrinol (Lausanne).* 2013;4:62.

26. Schwartz AV, et al. Diabetes and bone loss at the hip in older black and white adults. *J Bone Miner Res.* 2005;20:596-603.

27. Kuipers AL, et al. Renal function and bone loss in a cohort of Afro-Caribbean men. *J Bone Miner Res.* 2015;30:2215-20.

28. Stone KL, Bauer DC, Sellmeyer D, Cummings SR. Low serum vitamin B-12 levels are associated with increased hip bone loss in older women: A prospective study. *J Clin Endocrinol Metab.* 2004;89:1217-21.

29. Moayyeri A, Hammond CJ, Hart DJ, Spector TD. Effects of age on genetic influence on bone loss over 17 years in women: The Healthy Ageing Twin Study (HATS). *J Bone Miner Res.* 2012;27:2170-8.

30. Bauer DC, et al. Biochemical markers of bone turnover and prediction of hip bone loss in older women: The study of osteoporotic fractures. *J Bone Miner Res* 1999;14:1404-10.

31. Sellmeyer DE, Stone KL, Sebastian A, Cummings SR. A high ratio of dietary animal to vegetable protein increases the rate of bone loss and the risk of fracture in postmenopausal women. Study of Osteoporotic Fractures Research Group. *Am J Clin Nutr.* 2001;73:118-22.

32. Collins TC, et al. Peripheral arterial disease is associated with higher rates of hip bone loss and increased fracture risk in older men. *Circulation.* 2009;119:2305-12.

33. Tabatabai LS, et al. Arterialized venous bicarbonate is associated with lower bone mineral density and an increased rate of bone loss in older men and women. *J Clin Endocrinol Metab.* 2015;100:1343-9.

34. Sirola J, et al. Relation of statin use and bone loss: A prospective population-based cohort study in early postmenopausal women. *Osteoporos Int.* 2002;13:537-41.

35. Nakamura K, et al. Nutritional and biochemical parameters associated with 6-year change in bone mineral density in community-dwelling Japanese women aged 69 years and older: The Muramatsu Study. *Nutrition.* 2012;28:357-61.

36. Roy DK, et al. Determinants of incident vertebral fracture in men and women: Results from the European Prospective Osteoporosis Study (EPOS). *Osteoporos Int.* 2003;14:19-26.

37. Kanis JA, et al. Smoking and fracture risk: A meta-analysis. *Osteoporos Int.* 2005;16:155-62.

38. Cauley JA, et al. Risk factors for hip fracture in older men: The Osteoporotic Fractures in Men Study (MrOS). *J Bone Miner Res.* 2016. doi:10.1002/jbmr.2836.

39. Nevitt MC, et al. Risk factors for a first-incident radiographic vertebral fracture in women > or = 65 years of age: The study of osteoporotic fractures. *J Bone Miner Res.* 2005;20:131-40.

40. Cornuz J, Feskanich D, Willett WC, Colditz GA. Smoking, smoking cessation, and risk of hip fracture in women. *Am J Med.* 1999;106:311-4.

41. Thorin MH, Wihlborg A, Åkesson K, Gerdhem P. Smoking, smoking cessation, and fracture risk in elderly women followed for 10 years. *Osteoporos Int.* 2015;249-255. doi:10.1007/s00198-015-3290-z.

42. Mukamal KJ, Robbins JA, Cauley JA, Kern LM, Siscovick DS. Alcohol consumption, bone density, and hip fracture among older adults: The cardiovascular health study. *Osteoporos Int.* 2007;18:593-602.

43. Kubo JT, et al. Preference for wine is associated with lower hip fracture incidence in post-menopausal women. *BMC Womens Health.* 2013;13:36.

44. Compston JE, et al. Relationship of weight, height, and body mass index with fracture risk at different sites in postmenopausal women: The Global Longitudinal study of Osteoporosis in Women (GLOW). *J Bone Miner Res.* 2014;29:487-93.

45. Compston JE, et al. Obesity is not protective against fracture in post-menopausal women: GLOW. *Am J Med.* 2011;124:1043-50.

46. Compston JE, et al. Increase in fracture risk following unintentional weight loss in postmenopausal women: The Global Longitudinal Study of Osteoporosis in Women. *J Bone Miner Res.* 2016;31:1466-72.

47. FitzGerald G, et al. Differing risk profiles for individual fracture sites: Evidence from the Global Longitudinal Study of Osteoporosis in Women (GLOW). *J Bone Miner Res.* 2012;27:1907-15.

48. Lacombe J, et al. The effects of age, adiposity, and physical activity on the risk of seven site-specific fractures in postmenopausal women. *J Bone Miner Res.* 2016;31:1559-68.

49. Meyer HE, Willett WC, Flint AJ, Feskanich D. Abdominal obesity and hip fracture: Results from the Nurses' Health Study and the Health Professionals Follow-up Study. *Osteoporos Int.* 2016;27:2127-36.

50. Morseth B, et al. Leisure time physical activity and risk of non-vertebral fracture in men and women aged 55 years and older: The Tromsø Study. *Eur J Epidemiol.* 2012;27:463-71.

51. Kennedy CC, et al. A Frailty Index predicts 10-year fracture risk in adults age 25 years and older: Results from the Canadian Multicentre Osteoporosis Study (CaMos). *Osteoporos Int.* 2014;25:2825-32.

52. Ensrud KE, et al. A comparison of frailty indexes for the prediction of falls, disability, fractures, and mortality in older men. *J Am Geriatr Soc.* 2009;57:492-8.

53. Cawthon PM, et al. Physical performance and risk of hip fractures in older men. *J Bone Miner Res.* 2008;23:1037-44.

54. Barbour KE, et al. Trajectories of lower extremity physical performance: Effects on fractures and mortality in older women. *J Gerontol A Biol Sci Med Sci.* 2016. doi:10.1093/gerona/glw071.

55. Kärkkäinen M, et al. Association between functional capacity tests and fractures: An eight-year prospective population-based cohort study. *Osteoporos Int.* 2008;19:1203-10.

56. Kaptoge S, et al. Low BMD is less predictive than reported falls for future limb fractures in women across Europe: Results from the European Prospective Osteoporosis Study. *Bone.* 2005;36:387-398.

57. Wihlborg A, Englund M, Åkesson K, Gerdhem P. Fracture predictive ability of physical performance tests and history of falls in elderly women: A 10-year prospective study. *Osteoporos Int.* 2015;26:2101-9.

58. Thorell K, Ranstad K, Midlöv P, Borgquist L, Halling A. Is use of fall risk-increasing drugs in an elderly population associated with an increased risk of hip fracture, after adjustment for multimorbidity level: A cohort study. *BMC Geriatr.* 2014;14:131.

59. Stone KL, et al. Sleep disturbances and risk of falls in older community-dwelling men: The outcomes of Sleep Disorders in Older Men (MrOS Sleep) Study. *J Am Geriatr Soc.* 2014;62:299-305.

60. Gillespie LD, et al. Interventions for preventing falls in older people living in the community. *Cochrane Database Syst Rev.* 9, CD007146. 2012.

61. Nevitt MC, Cummings SR. Type of fall and risk of hip and wrist fractures: The study of osteoporotic fractures. The Study of Osteoporotic Fractures Research Group. *J Am Geriatr Soc.* 1993;41:1226-34.

62. Meier C, et al. Endogenous sex hormones and incident fracture risk in older men: The Dubbo Osteoporosis Epidemiology Study. *Arch Intern Med.* 2008;168:47-54.

63. Mellström D, et al. Older men with low serum estradiol and high serum SHBG have an increased risk of fractures. *J Bone Miner Res.* 2008;23:1552-60.

64. Mellström D, et al. Free testosterone is an independent predictor of BMD and prevalent fractures in elderly men: MrOS Sweden. *J Bone Miner Res.* 2006;21:529-35.

65. Barrett-Connor E, et al. The association of concurrent vitamin D and sex hormone deficiency with bone loss and fracture risk in older men: The MrOS study. *J Bone Miner Res.* 2012;27:2306-13.

66. Finigan J, et al. Endogenous estradiol and the risk of incident fracture in postmenopausal women: The OPUS study. *Calcif Tissue Int.* 2012;91:59-68.

67. Lim VW, et al. Serum free estradiol and estrogen receptor-α mediated activity are related to decreased incident hip fractures in older women. *Bone.* 2012;50:1311-6.

68. Ettinger B, et al. Associations between low levels of serum estradiol, bone density, and fractures among elderly women: The study of osteoporotic fractures. *J Clin Endocrinol Metab.* 1998;83:2239-43.

69. Cawthon PM, et al. Sex hormones, sex hormone binding globulin, and vertebral fractures in older men. *Bone.* 2016;84:271-8.

70. Fink HA, et al. Association of Parkinson's disease with accelerated bone loss, fractures and mortality in older men: The Osteoporotic Fractures in Men (MrOS) study. *Osteoporos Int.* 2008;19:1277-82.

71. Garin MC, Arnold AM, Lee JS, Robbins J, Cappola AR. Subclinical thyroid dysfunction and hip fracture and bone mineral density in older adults: The cardiovascular health study. *J Clin Endocrinol Metab.* 2014. 99:jc20141051.

72. Abrahamsen B, et al. Low serum thyrotropin level and duration of suppression as a predictor of major osteoporotic fractures – The OPENTHYRO register cohort. *J Bone Miner Res.* 2014;29:2040-50.

73. Blum MR, et al. Subclinical thyroid dysfunction and fracture risk. *JAMA.* 2015;313:2055.

74. Rosen CJ, et al. IOM Committee members respond to Endocrine Society Vitamin D Guideline. *J Clin Endocrinol Metab.* 2012;97:1146-52.

75. Fuleihan G, et al. Serum 25-Hydroxyvitamin D Levels: Variability, Knowledge Gaps, and the Concept of a Desirable Range. *J Bone Miner Res.* 2015;30:1119-33.

76. Cauley JA, et al. Serum 25-hydroxyvitamin D and clinical fracture risk in a multiethnic cohort of women: The Women's Health Initiative (WHI). *J Bone Miner Res.* 2011;26:2378-88.

77. Rejnmark L, Vestergaard P, Brot C, Mosekilde L. Increased fracture risk in normocalcemic postmenopausal women with high parathyroid hormone levels: A 16-year follow-up study. *Calcif Tissue Int.* 2011;88:238-45.

78. O'Sullivan S, Grey A. Adverse skeletal effects of drugs – Beyond glucocorticoids. *Clin Endocrinol (Oxf).* 2015;82:12-22.

79. Abrahamsen B, Brixen K. Mapping the prescriptiome to fractures in men – A national analysis of prescription history and fracture risk. *Osteoporos Int.* 2008;20:585-97.

80. De Vries F, et al. Fracture risk with intermittent high-dose oral glucocorticoid therapy. *Arthritis Rheum.* 2007;56:208-14.

81. van Staa TP, Leufkens HG, Abenhaim L, Zhang B, Cooper C. Oral corticosteroids and fracture risk: Relationship to daily and cumulative doses. *Rheumatology.* 2000;39:1383-9.

82. Abrahamsen B, et al. Fracture risk in Danish men with prostate cancer: A nationwide register study. *BJU Int.* 2007;100:749-54.

83. Lopez AM, et al. Fracture risk in patients with prostate cancer on androgen deprivation therapy. *Osteoporos Int.* 2005;16:707-11.

84. Rizzoli R, et al. Guidance for the prevention of bone loss and fractures in postmenopausal women treated with aromatase inhibitors for breast cancer: An ESCEO position paper. *Osteoporos Int.* 2012;23: 2567-76.

85. Abrahamsen B, et al. The excess risk of major osteoporotic fractures in hypothyroidism is driven by cumulative hyperthyroid as opposed to hypothyroid time: An observational register-based time-resolved cohort analysis. *J Bone Miner Res.* 2015;30:898-905.

86. Abrahamsen B, Vestergaard P. Proton pump inhibitor use and fracture risk – Effect modification by histamine H1 receptor blockade. Observational case-control study using National Prescription Data. *Bone.* 2013;57:269-71.

87. Andersen BN, Johansen PB, Abrahamsen B. Proton pump inhibitors and osteoporosis. *Curr Opin Rheumatol.* 2016;28:1.

88. Ngamruengphong S, Leontiadis GI, Radhi S, Dentino A, Nugent K. Proton pump inhibitors and risk of fracture: A systematic review and meta-analysis of observational studies. *Am J Gastroenterol.* 2011;106:1209-18; quiz 1219.

89. Souverein PC, Webb DJ, Weil JG, van Staa TP, Egberts AC. Use of anti-epileptic drugs and risk of fractures: Case-control study among patients with epilepsy. *Neurology.* 2006;66:1318-24.

90. Vestergaard P, Rejnmark L, Mosekilde L. Fracture risk associated with use of antiepileptic drugs. *Epilepsia.* 2004;45:1330-7.

91. Lunt M, et al. Characteristics of a prevalent vertebral deformity predict subsequent vertebral fracture: Results from the European Prospective Osteoporosis Study (EPOS). *Bone*. 2003;33:505-13.

92. Ismail AA, O'Neill TW, Cooper C, Silman AJ. Risk factors for vertebral deformities in men: Relationship to number of vertebral deformities. European Vertebral Osteoporosis Study Group. *J Bone Miner Res*. 2000;15:278-83.

93. Karlsson MK, et al. Characteristics of prevalent vertebral fractures predict new fractures in elderly men. *J Bone Joint Surg Am*. 2016;98:379-85.

94. McCloskey EV, Johansson H, Oden A, Kanis JA. From relative risk to absolute fracture risk calculation: The FRAX algorithm. *Curr Osteoporos Rep*. 2009;7:77-83.

95. Cummings SR, Melton LJ. Epidemiology and outcomes of osteoporotic fractures. *Lancet*. 2016;359:1761-7.

96. Naves M, Diaz-Lopez JB, Gomez C, Rodriguez-Rebollar A, Cannata-Andia JB. Determinants of incidence of osteoporotic fractures in the female Spanish population older than 50. *Osteoporos Int*. 2005;16:2013-7.

97. Scholes S, et al. Epidemiology of lifetime fracture prevalence in England: A population study of adults aged 55 years and over. *Age Ageing*. 2014;43:234-40.

98. Mosekilde L, Eriksen EF, Charles P. Effects of thyroid hormones on bone and mineral metabolism. *Endocrinol Metab Clin North Am*. 1990; 19:35-63.

99. Langdahl BL, et al. Bone mass, bone turnover, calcium homeostasis, and body composition in surgically and radioiodine-treated former hyperthyroid patients. *Thyroid*. 1996;6:169-75.

100. Gorka J, Taylor-Gjevre RM, Arnason T. Metabolic and clinical consequences of hyperthyroidism on bone density. *Int J Endocrinol*. 2013;2013:638727.

101. Mosekilde L, Melsen F. A tetracycline-based histomorphometric evaluation of bone resorption and bone turnover in hyperthyroidism and hyperparathyroidism. *Acta Med Scand*. 1978;204:97-102.

102. Vestergaard P, Mosekilde L, Hyperthyroidism, bone mineral, and fracture risk – A meta-analysis. *Thyroid*. 2003;13:585-93.

103. Starup-Linde J, Frost M, Vestergaard P, Abrahamsen B. Epidemiology of fractures in diabetes. *Calcif Tissue Int*. 2016. doi:10.1007/s00223-016 -0175-x.

104. Fraser L-A, Papaioannou A, Adachi JD, Ma J, Thabane L. Fractures are increased and bisphosphonate use decreased in individuals with insulin-dependent diabetes: A 10 year cohort study. *BMC Musculoskelet Disord*. 2014;15:201.

105. Vestergaard P, Rejnmark L, Mosekilde L. Diabetes and its complications and their relationship with risk of fractures in type 1 and 2 diabetes. *Calcif Tissue Int*. 2009;84:45-55.

106. Napoli N, et al. Mechanisms of diabetes mellitus-induced bone fragility. *Nat Rev Endocrinol*. 2016. doi:10.1038/nrendo.2016.153.

107. Hansen D, Olesen JB, Gislason GH, Abrahamsen B, Hommel K. Risk of fracture in adults on renal replacement therapy: A Danish national cohort study. *Nephrol Dial Transplant*. gfw073. 2016. doi:10.1093/ndt /gfw073.

108. Ensrud KE, et al. Estimated GFR and risk of hip fracture in older men: Comparison of associations using cystatin C and creatinine. *Am J Kidney Dis*. 2014;63:31-9.

109. Ensrud KE, et al. Renal function and nonvertebral fracture risk in multi-ethnic women: The Women's Health Initiative (WHI). *Osteoporos Int*. 2012;23:887-99.

110. Premaor MO, et al. Fracture incidence after liver transplantation: Results of a 10-year audit. *QJM*. 2011;104:599-606.

111. Sprague SM, Josephson MA. Bone disease after kidney transplantation. *Semin Nephrol*. 2004;24:82-90.

112. Vestergaard P, Mosekilde L. Fractures in patients with primary hyperpara-thyroidism: Nationwide follow-up study of 1201 patients. *World J Surg*. 2003;27:343-9.

113. Card T, West J, Hubbard R, Logan RF. Hip fractures in patients with inflammatory bowel disease and their relationship to corticosteroid use: A population based cohort study. *Gut*. 2004;53:251-5.

114. Targownik LE, et al. Inflammatory bowel disease and the risk of fracture after controlling for FRAX. *J Bone Miner Res*. 2013;28:1007-13.

115. Vázquez MA, et al. Vertebral fractures in patients with inflammatory bowel disease compared with a healthy population: A prospective case-control study. *BMC Gastroenterol*. 2012;12:47.

116. Heikkila K, et al. Celiac disease autoimmunity and hip fracture risk: Findings from a prospective cohort study. *J Bone Miner Res*. 2015;30:630-6.

117. Olmos M, et al. Systematic review and meta-analysis of observational studies on the prevalence of fractures in coeliac disease. *Dig Liver Dis*. 2008;40:46-53.

118. Vestergaard P, et al. Fractures in patients with anorexia nervosa, bulimia nervosa, and other eating disorders – A nationwide register study. *Int J Eat Disord*. 2002;32:301-8.

119. Howgate DJ, et al. Bone metabolism in anorexia nervosa: Molecular pathways and current treatment modalities. *Osteoporos Int*. 2013;24:407-21.

120. Misra M, Golden NH, Katzman DK. State of the art systematic review of bone disease in anorexia nervosa. *Int J Eat Disord*. 2016;49:276-92.

121. Sullivan SD, et al. Effects of self-reported age at nonsurgical menopause on time to first fracture and bone mineral density in the Women's Health Initiative Observational Study. *Menopause*. 2015;22:1035-44.

122. Kim SY, et al. Risk of osteoporotic fracture in a large population-based cohort of patients with rheumatoid arthritis. *Arthritis Res Ther*. 2010;12:R154.

123. Amin S, Gabriel SE, Achenbach SJ, Atkinso, EJ, Melton LJ. Are young women and men with rheumatoid arthritis at risk for fragility fractures? A population-based study. *J Rheumatol*. 2013;40:1669-76.

124. Dennison EM, et al. Is allopurinol use associated with an excess risk of osteoporotic fracture? A National Prescription Registry study. *Arch Osteoporos.* 2015;10:36.

125. Basu U, et al. Association between allopurinol use and hip fracture in older patients. *Bone.* 2016;84:189-93.

126. Kim SC, Paik JM, Liu J, Curhan GC, Solomon DH. Gout and the risk of non-vertebral fracture. *J Bone Miner Res.* 2016. doi:10.1002/jbmr.2978.

127. Muka T, et al. The Influence of Serum Uric Acid on Bone Mineral Density, Hip Geometry, and Fracture Risk: The Rotterdam Study. *J Clin Endocrinol Metab.* 2016;101:1113-22.

128. Lane NE, et al. Association of serum uric acid and incident nonspine fractures in elderly men: The Osteoporotic Fractures in Men (MrOS) Study. *J Bone Miner Res.* 2014;29:1701-7.

129. Lustberg MB, Reinbolt RE, Shapiro CL. Bone health in adult cancer survivorship. *J Clin Oncol.* 2012;30:3665-74.

130. Rousseau C, et al. Change in fracture risk and fracture pattern after bariatric surgery: Nested case-control study. *BMJ.* 2016;354:i3794.

131. Langsetmo L, et al. Associations of Protein Intake and Protein Source with Bone Mineral Density and Fracture Risk: A Population-Based Cohort Study. *J Nutr Health Aging.* 2015;19:861-8.

132. Ioannidis G, et al. Glucocorticoids predict 10-year fragility fracture risk in a population-based ambulatory cohort of men and women: Canadian Multicentre Osteoporosis Study (CaMos). *Arch Osteoporos.* 2014;9:169.

133. Papaioannou A, et al. Risk factors associated with incident clinical vertebral and nonvertebral fractures in postmenopausal women: The Canadian Multicentre Osteoporosis Study (CaMos). *Osteoporos Int.* 2005;16, 568-78.

134. Barzilay JI, et al. Albuminuria is associated with hip fracture risk in older adults: The Cardiovascular Health Study. *Osteoporos Int.* 2013;24:2993–3000.

135. Carbone L, et al. Hip fractures and heart failure: Findings from the Cardiovascular Health Study. *Eur Heart J.* 2010;31:77-84.

136. Bethel M, et al. Soluble CD14 and fracture risk. *Osteoporos Int.* 2016;27:1755-63.

137. Barzilay JI, et al. Fibrosis markers, hip fracture risk, and bone density in older adults. *Osteoporos Int.* 2016;27:815-20.

138. Rejnmark L, et al. Fracture risk in perimenopausal women treated with beta-blockers. *Calcif Tissue Int.* 2004;75:365-72.

139. Vestergaard P, Hermann P, Jensen J-EB, Eiken P, Mosekilde L. Effects of paracetamol, non-steroidal anti-inflammatory drugs, acetylsalicylic acid, and opioids on bone mineral density and risk of fracture: Results of the Danish Osteoporosis Prevention Study (DOPS). *Osteoporos Int.* 2012;23: 1255-65.

140. Chan MY, Center JR, Eisman JA, Nguyen TV. Bone mineral density and association of osteoarthritis with fracture risk. *Osteoarthritis Cartilage.* 2014;22:1251-8.

141. Yang S, Nguyen ND, Center JR, Eisman JA, Nguyen TV. Association between hypertension and fragility fracture: A longitudinal study. *Osteoporos Int.* 2014;25:97-103.

142. Yang S, et al. Association between beta-blocker use and fracture risk: The Dubbo Osteoporosis Epidemiology Study. *Bone.* 2011;48:451-5.

143. Vesco KK, et al. Surgical menopause and nonvertebral fracture risk among older US women. *Menopause.* 2012;19:510-6.

144. Hayhoe RPG, Lentjes MAH, Luben RN, Khaw K-T, Welch AA. Dietary magnesium and potassium intakes and circulating magnesium are associated with heel bone ultrasound attenuation and osteoporotic fracture risk in the EPIC-Norfolk cohort study. *Am J Clin Nutr.* 2015;102:376-84.

145. Hannan MT, et al. Height loss predicts subsequent hip fracture in men and women of the Framingham Study. *J Bone Miner Res.* 2012;27:146-52.

146. Sahni S, et al. Protective effect of total and supplemental vitamin C intake on the risk of hip fracture – A 17-year follow-up from the Framingham Osteoporosis Study. *Osteoporos Int.* 2009;20:1853-61.

147. McLean RR, et al. Homocysteine as a predictive factor for hip fracture in older persons. *N Engl J Med.* 2004;350:2042-9.

148. Kiel DP, Felson DT, Hannan MT, Anderson JJ, Wilson PW. Caffeine and the risk of hip fracture: The Framingham Study. *Am J Epidemiol.* 1990; 132:675-84.

149. Williams LJ, et al. Depression as a risk factor for fracture in women: A 10 year longitudinal study. *J Affect Disord.* 2016;192:34-40.

150. Pasco JA, et al. Beta-adrenergic blockers reduce the risk of fracture partly by increasing bone mineral density: Geelong Osteoporosis Study. *J Bone Miner Res.* 2004;19:19-24.

151. Sanders KM, et al. Fracture rates lower in rural than urban communities: The Geelong Osteoporosis Study. *J Epidemiol Commun Health.* 2002; 56:466-70.

152. Kärkkäinen M, et al. Association between functional capacity tests and fractures: An eight-year prospective population-based cohort study. *Osteoporos Int.* 2008;19:1203-10.

153. Honkanen R, Tuppurainen M, Kröger H, Alhava E, Saarikoski S. Relationships between risk factors and fractures differ by type of fracture: A population-based study of 12,192 perimenopausal women. *Osteoporos Int.* 1998; 8:25-31.

154. Armstrong ME, et al. Relationship of height to site-specific fracture risk in postmenopausal women. *J Bone Miner Res.* 2016;31:725-31.

155. Meisinger C, Heier M, Lang O, Döring A. Beta-blocker use and risk of fractures in men and women from the general population: The MONICA/KORA Augsburg cohort study. *Osteoporos Int.* 2007;18:1189-95.

156. Jamal SA, et al. Hyponatremia and fractures: Findings from the MrOS Study. *J Bone Miner Res.* 2015;30:970-5.

157. Lewerin C, et al. Low holotranscobalamin and cobalamins predict incident fractures in elderly men: The MrOS Sweden. *Osteoporos Int.* 2014;25:131-40.

158. Barrett-Connor E, et al. The association of concurrent vitamin D and sex hormone deficiency with bone loss and fracture risk in older men: The MrOS study. *J Bone Miner Res.* 2012. doi:10.1002/jbmr.1697.

159. Sheu Y, et al. Abdominal body composition measured by quantitative computed tomography and risk of non-spine fractures: The Osteoporotic Fractures in Men (MrOS) Study. *Osteoporos Int.* 2013;24:2231-41.

160. Yu R, Leung J, Woo J. Incremental predictive value of sarcopenia for incident fracture in an elderly Chinese cohort: Results from the Osteoporotic Fractures in Men (MrOs) Study. *J Am Med Dir Assoc.* 2014;15:551-8.

161. Waring AC, et al. A prospective study of thyroid function, bone loss, and fractures in older men: The MrOS study. *J Bone Miner Res.* 2013; 28:472-9.

162. Nielson CM, et al. BMI and fracture risk in older men: The Osteoporotic Fractures in Men Study (MrOS). *J Bone Miner Res.* 2011;26:496-502.

163. Faulkner KA, et al. Histories including number of falls may improve risk prediction for certain non-vertebral fractures in older men. *Inj Prev.* 2009;15:307-11.

164. Cauley JA, et al. Inflammatory markers and the risk of hip and vertebral fractures in men: The Osteoporotic Fractures in Men (MrOS). *J Bone Miner Res.* 2016. doi:10.1002/jbmr.2905.

165. Wallin M, et al. Low-level cadmium exposure is associated with decreased bone mineral density and increased risk of incident fractures in elderly men: The MrOS Sweden Study. *J Bone Miner Res.* 2016;31:732-41.

166. Cawthon PM, et al. Change in hip bone mineral density and risk of subsequent fractures in older men. *J Bone Miner Res.* 2012;27:2179-88.

167. Johansson H, et al. Waning predictive value of serum adiponectin for fracture risk in elderly men: MrOS Sweden. *Osteoporos Int.* 2014. doi:10.1007 /s00198-014-2654-0.

168. Szulc P, et al. High hip fracture risk in men with severe aortic calcification: MrOS study. *J Bone Miner Res.* 2014;29:968-75.

169. Mirza MA, et al. Serum fibroblast growth factor-23 (FGF-23) and fracture risk in elderly men. *J Bone Miner Res.* 2011;26:857-64.

170. Tanaka S, et al. Serum 25-hydroxyvitamin D below 25 ng/mL is a risk factor for long bone fracture comparable to bone mineral density in Japanese postmenopausal women. *J Bone Miner Metab.* 2014;32:514-23.

171. Looker AC. Hemoglobin and hip fracture risk in older non-Hispanic white adults. *Osteoporos Int.* 2014;25:2389-98.

172. Finnes TE, et al. A combination of low serum concentrations of vitamins K1 and D is associated with increased risk of hip fractures in elderly Norwegians: A NOREPOS study. *Osteoporos Int.* 2016;27:1645-52.

173. Paik JM, Rosen HN, Gordon CM, Curhan GC. diuretic use and risk of vertebral fracture in women. *Am J Med.* 2016. doi:10.1016/j.amjmed .2016.07.013.

174. Feskanich D, Hankinson SE, Schernhammer ES. Nightshift work and fracture risk: The Nurses' Health Study. *Osteoporos Int.* 2009;20: 537-42.

175. Fung TT, Feskanich D. Dietary patterns and risk of hip fractures in post-menopausal women and men over 50 years. *Osteoporos Int*. 2015;26: 1825-30.

176. Fung TT, et al. Soda consumption and risk of hip fractures in postmeno-pausal women in the Nurses' Health Study. *Am J Clin Nutr*. 2014;100:953-8.

177. Yang S, Feskanich D, Willett WC, Eliassen AH, Wu T. Association between global biomarkers of oxidative stress and hip fracture in postmenopausal women: A prospective study. *J Bone Miner Res*. 2014;29:2577-83.

178. Périer MA, Gineyts E, Munoz F, Sornay-Rendu E, Delmas PD. Homocysteine and fracture risk in postmenopausal women: The OFELY study. *Osteoporos Int*. 2007;18:1329-36.

179. Roux JP, Belghali S, Wegrzyn J, Rendu ES, Chapurlat R. Vertebral body morphology is associated with incident lumbar vertebral fracture in post-menopausal women. The OFELY study. *Osteoporos Int*. 2016;27:2507-13.

180. Rousseau JC, Sornay-Rendu E, Bertholon C, Chapurlat R, Garnero P. Serum periostin is associated with fracture risk in postmenopausal women: A 7-year prospective analysis of the OFELY study. *J Clin Endocrinol Metab*. 2014;99:2533-9.

181. Goerss JB, et al. Risk of fractures in patients with pernicious anemia. *J Bone Min Res*. 1992;7:573-9.

182. Melton LJ, Atkinson EJ, O'Fallon WM, Heath, H. Risk of age-related fractures in patients with primary hyperparathyroidism. *Arch Intern Med*. 1992;152:2269-73.

183. Cooper C, et al. Fracture risk in patients with ankylosing spondylitis: A population based study. *J Rheumatol*. 1994;21:1877-82.

184. de Jonge EAL, et al. Dietary vitamin A intake and bone health in the elderly: The Rotterdam Study. *Eur J Clin Nutr*. 2015;69:1360-8.

185. Hoorn EJ, et al. Mild hyponatremia as a risk factor for fractures: The Rotterdam Study. *J Bone Miner Res*. 2011;26:1822-8.

186. Yazdanpanah N, et al. Effect of dietary B vitamins on BMD and risk of fracture in elderly men and women: The Rotterdam study. *Bone*. 2007; 41:987-94.

187. van der Deure WM, et al. Effects of serum TSH and FT4 levels and the TSHR-Asp727Glu polymorphism on bone: The Rotterdam Study. *Clin Endocrinol (Oxf)*. 2008;68:175-81.

188. van Meurs JBJ, et al. Homocysteine levels and the risk of osteoporotic fracture. *N Engl J Med*. 2004;350:2033-41.

189. Castaño-Betancourt MC, et al. Association of lumbar disc degeneration with osteoporotic fractures; the Rotterdam study and meta-analysis from systematic review. *Bone*. 2013;57:284-9.

190. Goderie-Plomp HW, et al. Endogenous sex hormones, sex hormone-binding globulin, and the risk of incident vertebral fractures in elderly men and women: The Rotterdam Study. *J Clin Endocrinol Metab*. 2004;89:3261-9.

191. Dai Z, et al. Protective effects of dietary carotenoids on risk of hip fracture in men: The Singapore Chinese Health Study. *J Bone Miner Res.* 2014;29:408-17.

192. Koh W-P, et al. Gender-specific associations between soy and risk of hip fracture in the Singapore Chinese Health Study. *Am J Epidemiol.* 2009;170:901-9.

193. Coleman AL, et al. Visual field loss and risk of fractures in older women. *J Am Geriatr Soc.* 2009;57:1825-32.

194. Michaëlsson K, Wolk A, Byberg L, Ärnlöv J, Melhus H. Intake and serum concentrations of α-tocopherol in relation to fractures in elderly women and men: 2 cohort studies. *Am J Clin Nutr.* 2014;99:107-14.

195. Byberg L, Bellavia A, Orsini N, Wolk A, Michaëlsson K. Fruit and vegetable intake and risk of hip fracture: A cohort study of Swedish men and women. *J Bone Miner Res.* 2015;30:976-84.

196. Snellman G, et al. Long-term dietary vitamin D intake and risk of fracture and osteoporosis: A longitudinal cohort study of Swedish middle-aged and elderly women. *J Clin Endocrinol Metab.* 2014;99:781-90.

197. Jørgensen L, Joakimsen R, Ahmed L, Størmer J, Jacobsen BK. Smoking is a strong risk factor for non-vertebral fractures in women with diabetes: The Tromsø Study. *Osteoporos Int.* 2011;22:1247-53.

198. Ahmed LA, Schirmer H, Berntsen GK, Fønnebø V, Joakimsen RM. Self-reported diseases and the risk of non-vertebral fractures: The Tromsø study. *Osteoporos Int.* 2006;17:46-53.

199. Joakimsen RM, Fønnebø V, Magnus JH, Tollan A, Søgaard AJ. The Tromsø Study: Body height, body mass index and fractures. *Osteoporos Int.* 1998;8:436-42.

200. Chen Z, et al. The relationship between incidence of fractures and anemia in older multiethnic women. *J Am Geriatr Soc.* 2010;58:2337-44.

201. Orchard TS, et al. Fatty acid consumption and risk of fracture in the Women's Health Initiative. *Am J Clin Nutr.* 2010;92:1452-60.

202. Spangler L, et al. Depressive symptoms, bone loss, and fractures in post-menopausal women. *J Gen Intern Med.* 2008;23:567-74.

203. Carbone LD, et al. Urinary Tract Stones and Osteoporosis: Findings From the Women's Health Initiative. *J Bone Miner Res.* 2015;30:2096-102.

204. Crandall CJ, et al. Associations of menopausal vasomotor symptoms with fracture incidence. *J Clin Endocrinol Metab.* 2015;100:524-34.

205. LaCroix AZ, et al. OPG and sRANKL serum levels and incident hip fracture in postmenopausal Caucasian women in the Women's Health Initiative Observational Study. *Bone.* 2013;56:474-81.

11

Risk factors for post peak bone loss and osteoporotic fracture: Lessons from novel imaging studies

NAMRATA MADHUSUDAN, MARK H EDWARDS
AND ELAINE M DENNISON

INTRODUCTION

In an ageing population, osteoporosis represents a major and ever increasing burden of disease, with great personal, societal and economic consequences following associated fragility fractures. Against this background, developments in the identification and investigation of patients with osteoporosis and at risk of fracture are becoming ever more important.

The current international gold standard for identification of patients with low bone mass is dual-energy X-ray absorptiometry (DXA) (1). While there have been great advances in areal bone mineral density (aBMD) measurement in recent years, there are well-identified limitations with DXA. DXA is a two-dimensional imaging modality, and is unable to distinguish between trabecular and cortical bone (2). It has very limited capacity to make assessments of bone geometry, and it is becoming increasingly evident that microarchitectural changes in bone composition play a fundamental role in bone health, and subsequently fracture risk. It also fails to give information on volumetric bone mineral density (vBMD) (3).

In recent years, novel cross-sectional imaging techniques have been employed in a research setting to improve understanding of the determinants of fracture risk in patients with osteoporosis. One such technique is high-resolution peripheral quantitative computed tomography (HRpQCT) (3). In this chapter, the role of HRpQCT in identification and assessment of risk factors for osteoporotic fractures is explored. For a detailed exposition of variation in bone indices by age and sex, the reader is referred to Chapter 9.

HIGH RESOLUTION PERIPHERAL COMPUTED TOMOGRAPHY

With the advent of high resolution, site-specific imaging techniques, HRpQCT has become an invaluable novel method of investigating bone microstructure at the peripheral skeleton. At present, there is only one commercially available extremity scanner (XtremeCT, Scanco Medical, Bruttisellen, Switzerland). Scans are acquired from standard imaging regions, at the ultradistal radius (proximal to the radiocarpal joint) and the ultradistal tibia (proximal to the ankle) (4). The wrist or ankle are immobilised within the scan gantry, which houses a fixed carbon cast (5). The operator uses a projection image to mark a reference line at the radial or tibial midjoint, from which the region of interest can be delineated (9.5 mm proximal to the radial reference line and 22.5 mm proximal to the tibial reference line). This can be modified in children and adolescents to avoid radiation exposure to the epiphyseal plate (5). A stack of two-dimensional grey-scale images is then reconstructed, using raw projection data acquired by the scanner (5). Images with an isotropic voxel size of 82 µm (110 slices, 9 mm scan length) (4) are produced, enabling delineation of bone microarchitecture, and by segmenting the regions, trabecular and cortical compartments can be separately studied (5) (Figure 11.1).

HRpQCT confers a number of advantages over conventional imaging techniques. It is a non-invasive imaging modality, with a rapid scan time of 2.8 minutes (5). HRpQCT provides high-resolution three-dimensional images of overall and compartment-specific bony microarchitecture (4), which previously required invasive transiliac bone biopsies (5). As only particular regions are targeted, there is a focused area of peripheral radiation exposure. To contextualise this level of radiation exposure, a patient undergoing a clinical abdominal CT scan is exposed to approximately a 500- to 1000-fold greater radiation dose. However, it must be remembered that HRpQCT is limited to distal peripheral sites such as the tibia and radius. As vertebral and hip fractures confer a significant burden of disease in osteoporosis, this is a major limitation of HRpQCT. It is also only possible to quantify mineralised bone, therefore mineralisation defects such as osteomalacia cannot be investigated (4).

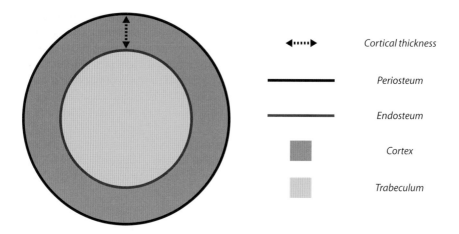

Figure 11.1 Cross-sectional representation of a tubular bone.

Despite its limitations, HRpQCT is becoming an increasingly popular method of investigating risk factors for post peak bone loss and osteoporotic fractures, with an emphasis on bone microarchitecture.

BODY COMPOSITION

It was estimated in 2014 that over 1.9 billion adults globally were overweight, of whom 600 million are classified as obese (6). It is a pervasive problem which affects all age groups, and it is therefore becoming increasingly important to further understand the relationship between body composition and body mass index (BMI) on bone health. HRpQCT has been used to investigate these associations.

In recent years, it has been shown that the relationship between adiposity and fracture risk is complex, being site specific and modified by BMD (7–9). In addition, overweight children have been shown to sustain more fractures in comparison to healthy weight children (10,11). In 2012 Hoy et al. (12) categorised male and female patients with a mean age of 17 and 18 years, respectively, into healthy and overweight groups, and used HRpQCT to investigate bone quality at the distal radius and tibia. They demonstrated that overweight males (BMI over 25 kg/m²) had higher trabecular volumetric BMD and number than healthy weight males (BMI under 25 kg/m²) at both sites. This difference in bone quality was attenuated by lean mass. In comparison, differences were not seen between overweight and healthy-weight females, suggesting that the relationship between bone architecture and BMI may be sex-specific, and affected by lean mass.

When comparing obese to matched control normal-weight adults, obese adults have been shown to have significantly greater vBMD at the distal tibia in younger (25–40 years) and older (55–75 years) adults, and at the distal radius in older adults. Younger obese adults also had greater trabecular density, and a greater cortical and trabecular density was seen in older obese adults. Bone size, however, did not differ at the radius or tibia (8).

Similarly, in obese men and premenopausal women with metabolic syndrome, HRpQCT was used to show correlations between lean mass and BMD of the total femur and radius, with no significant association between BMD and fat mass. In addition, lean mass was shown to be an independent factor influencing most HRpQCT variables, with trabecular vBMD and the ratio of trabecular bone volume to tissue volume only correlating in men (7). These studies hence suggest that lean mass plays an important role in bone quality and microarchitecture, as assessed by HRpQCT.

These data suggest that while obesity is associated with increased bone density when compared to healthy-weight adults, other factors including lean mass, sex and age are important when considering ultimate relationships with microarchitecture and fracture risk.

DIABETES

There are important sequelae associated with diabetes mellitus, including adverse effects on bone health. Patients with type 2 diabetes mellitus (T2DM) have a higher fracture risk compared to non-diabetic controls for a given femoral neck BMD T-score, age or FRAX probability (13). As diabetes mellitus is an independent risk factor for both central and peripheral fragility fractures, it is important to further understand the relationships between diabetes and bone health (14).

While current data are inconsistent, with the majority of studies in women, there is now evidence to suggest that cortical microarchitecture may play a role in fracture risk of patients with diabetes. A pilot cross-sectional study in 2010 used HRpQCT to characterise cortical and trabecular microarchitecture and biomechanics in postmenopausal women with T2DM (15). Volumetric index of cortical porosity and cortical pore volume were significantly higher in the radius of patients with T2DM compared to controls. A similar but non-significant trend was seen at the tibia. In addition, the vBMD at the distal tibia was significantly higher in patients with T2DM, mainly due to a 10% greater trabecular density adjacent to the cortex.

This was also demonstrated by HRpQCT in a cross-sectional case-control study of postmenopausal women with T2DM who had sustained fragility fractures, compared to T2DM non-fracture controls (16). At the ultradistal and distal tibia, diabetic patients with previous fractures were found to have a significantly higher intracortical pore volume and relative porosity compared to diabetic patients without fracture history. Intracortical pore volume was also significantly greater at the distal and ultradistal radius, with distal radial relative cortical porosity showing a similar significant trend.

Until recently, the relationship between bone microarchitecture and diabetes in men has been under-investigated. In 2016, Paccou et al. (14) studied this association in a cohort of diabetic men and women compared to controls without T2DM. Using HRpQCT, they demonstrated that diabetic men had a significantly greater cortical porosity and cortical pore volume and lower cortical vBMD at both tibia and radius compared to non-diabetic controls. They also demonstrated a significantly higher trabecular number at both the radius and tibia in diabetic men. Diabetic women were shown to have a significantly higher cortical porosity and cortical pore volume at the radius.

As cortical microarchitecture plays an important role in the initiation and propagation of fractures when subjected to bending loads, the changes in cortical volume and porosity may provide a possible explanation for increased fracture risk in diabetes. This may be coupled with a change in distribution of trabecular density and volume, as demonstrated by Burghardt et al. (15), furthering the propensity to fractures in diabetes.

SMOKING AND ALCOHOL

Alcohol

Results from previous studies have suggested that there is a dose-dependent relationship between levels of alcohol consumed and bone health, with low levels of alcohol consumption (between 0.5 and 1.0 unit per day) associated with a lower risk of hip fracture compared to abstainers and high alcohol intake (17). In addition, DXA has been used to show that there is a positive association between moderate alcohol intake and aBMD (18,19).

However, further investigation of geometric, volumetric and microarchitectural bone composition using HRpQCT has suggested a different pattern of association. In 2015, Paccou et al. (20) showed that at the distal radius in men, those who drank low levels (between 1 and <11 units per week) had lower cortical thickness, cortical vBMD and trabecular vBMD, and higher trabecular separation compared to those who drank minimal/no alcohol (less than 1 unit per week). Similar significant associations were seen in cortical microarchitecture in those with moderate to high alcohol consumption (11 or more units per week) when compared to individuals with no or minimal alcohol intake. In women, similar associations were demonstrated in those with low levels of alcohol consumption compared to minimal/no alcohol, with lower trabecular vBMD at the tibia reaching statistical significance. However, distal radial trabecular vBMD, trabecular thickness, trabecular number and trabecular separation were significantly higher in moderate/high levels of alcohol intake compared to in those who drank low alcohol. The difference in microarchitecture might be explained by the fact that DXA is affected by other variables such as body composition (20), whereas HRpQCT is not. Further investigation into this association is required.

Smoking

It has been shown that smoking results in a significantly lower aBMD as demonstrated by DXA, and lower cortical radial and tibial thickness as seen on peripheral quantitative CT (21). However, there are limited data on the relationship between bone microarchitecture and smoking, as investigated by HRpQCT. Longitudinal follow-up of a cohort by Rudang et al. (22) documented a significantly lower tibial trabecular vBMD in smokers compared to non-smokers. Tibial trabecular bone

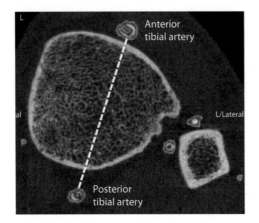

Figure 11.2 Lower leg arterial calcification. (Reproduced with permission from Paccou J et al. *Osteoporos Int*. 2016 Nov;27(11):3279-87.)

volume fraction was also significant in smokers. Importantly, lower limb arterial calcification in women has been associated with lower quality bone microstructure, as assessed by HRpQCT (Figure 11.2) (23).

FRACTURES

The assessment of bone health is clinically important in the context of identifying osteoporotic patients at high risk of fracture. While aBMD as measured by DXA is important in predicting fracture risk (24), it has been recognised that only approximately half of all fractures in postmenopausal women occur in those with an aBMD that falls below the WHO threshold for osteoporosis (25,26). Novel methods of bone health measurement, and consequently risk fracture prediction, are therefore increasingly important.

Through the use of HRpQCT, there has been a greater understanding that osteoporosis is a microarchitecturally diverse disease, with different bone phenotypes conferring variable levels of fracture risk (3). Edwards et al. (3) recently used HRpQCT to identify discrete patterns associated with fracture, each with varying bone geometry and microarchitectural structure, in a cohort of men and women recruited from the Hertfordshire Cohort Study. The authors demonstrated two high-risk bone phenotypes associated with fracture in both men and women, the first showing low cortical thickness and density, with a higher total and trabecular area in men. The second showed lower trabecular density and number in both sexes. In an unadjusted analysis, the odds of fracture were significantly higher in patients with lower cortical thickness. In women, a lower trabecular density, thickness and number also conferred greater odds of a prevalent fracture. In addition, these results were correlated with aBMD measurements obtained by DXA. Importantly, in those with lower cortical thickness, a smaller proportion of patients were shown to be osteoporotic according to their

DXA results. Men in this group also showed statistically nonsignificant differences in aBMD compared to a reference cluster. As cross-sectional bone size in men in this high-risk group of patients was larger, it is likely that the DXA results falsely elevated their aBMD results and were not accurately representative of their volumetric bone mineral density. This therefore suggests that if relying on DXA alone, an important group of patients at high risk for osteoporotic fractures would not be identified.

These results mirror previous studies on the relationship between bone microarchitecture and fracture. Case control studies have shown that both vertebral and nonvertebral fractures are associated with reduced bone mineral density in postmenopausal women. There is also evidence to suggest that there is an association between altered microarchitecture of both cortical and trabecular structure and osteoporotic fragility fractures, and these changes are only partially demonstrated by DXA aBMD (27–29).

CONCLUSION

HRpQCT can thus be used in the assessment of bone microarchitecture in the context of risk factors for post peak bone loss and osteoporotic fractures. There is an increasing body of evidence to suggest that the detailed images and measurements of bone microarchitecture provided are clinically meaningful and might contribute to risk assessment algorithms. However, in order for it to be incorporated into routine clinical practice, independence of the measurements from BMD and current risk assessment indices such as FRAX and robust risk prediction across large prospective cohorts would ideally be required.

REFERENCES

1. Popp AW, Windolf M, Senn C, Tami A, Richards RG, Brianza S, et al. Prediction of bone strength at the distal tibia by HR-pQCT and DXA. *Bone.* 2012 Jan;50(1):296-300. PubMed PMID: 22088678.
2. Pisani P, Renna MD, Conversano F, Casciaro E, Di Paola M, Quarta E, et al. Major osteoporotic fragility fractures: Risk factor updates and societal impact. *World J Orthop.* 2016 Mar 18;7(3):171-81. PubMed PMID: 27004165. PubMed Central PMCID: PMC4794536.
3. Edwards MH, Robinson DE, Ward KA, Javaid MK, Walker-Bone K, Cooper C, et al. Cluster analysis of bone microarchitecture from high resolution peripheral quantitative computed tomography demonstrates two separate phenotypes associated with high fracture risk in men and women. *Bone.* 2016 Jul;88:131-7. PubMed PMID: 27130873. PubMed Central PMCID: PMC4913839. Epub 2016/05/01. eng.
4. Patsch JM, Burghardt AJ, Kazakia G, Majumdar S. Noninvasive imaging of bone microarchitecture. *Ann N Y Acad Sci.* 2011 Dec;1240:77-87. PubMed PMID: 22172043. PubMed Central PMCID: PMC4461066.

5. Nishiyama KK, Shane E. Clinical imaging of bone microarchitecture with HR-pQCT. *Curr Osteoporos Rep.* 2013 Jun;11(2):147-55. PubMed PMID: 23504496. PubMed Central PMCID: PMC4102136.

6. Obesity and Overweight; fact sheet No 311. http://www.who.int /mediacentre/factsheets/fs311/en/2015. Cited 2016 June 20.

7. Madeira E, Mafort TT, Madeira M, Guedes EP, Moreira RO, de Mendonca LM, et al. Lean mass as a predictor of bone density and microarchitecture in adult obese individuals with metabolic syndrome. *Bone.* 2014 Feb;59:89-92. PubMed PMID: 24220493.

8. Evans AL, Paggiosi MA, Eastell R, Walsh JS. Bone density, microstructure and strength in obese and normal weight men and women in younger and older adulthood. *J Bone Miner Res.* 2015 May;30(5):920-8. PubMed PMID: 25400253.

9. Johansson H, Kanis JA, Oden A, McCloskey E, Chapurlat RD, Christiansen C, et al. A meta-analysis of the association of fracture risk and body mass index in women. *J Bone Miner Res.* 2014 Jan;29(1):223-33. PubMed PMID: 23775829. Epub 2013/06/19. eng.

10. Hills AP, Andersen LB, Byrne NM. Physical activity and obesity in children. *Br J Sports Med.* 2011 Sep;45(11):866-70. PubMed PMID: 21836171.

11. Taylor ED, Theim KR, Mirch MC, Ghorbani S, Tanofsky-Kraff M, Adler-Wailes DC, et al. Orthopedic complications of overweight in children and adolescents. *Pediatrics.* 2006 Jun;117(6):2167-74. PubMed PMID: 16740861. PubMed Central PMCID: PMC1863007.

12. Hoy CL, Macdonald HM, McKay HA. How does bone quality differ between healthy-weight and overweight adolescents and young adults? *Clin Orthop Relat Res.* 2013 Apr;471(4):1214-25. PubMed PMID: 23001501. PubMed Central PMCID: PMC3586045.

13. Schwartz AV, Vittinghoff E, Bauer DC, Hillier TA, Strotmeyer ES, Ensrud KE, et al. Association of BMD and FRAX score with risk of fracture in older adults with type 2 diabetes. *JAMA.* 2011 Jun 1;305(21):2184-92. PubMed PMID: 21632482. PubMed Central PMCID: PMC3287389.

14. Paccou J, Ward KA, Jameson KA, Dennison EM, Cooper C, Edwards MH. Bone microarchitecture in men and women with diabetes: The importance of cortical porosity. *Calcif Tissue Int.* 2016 May;98(5):465-73. PubMed PMID: 26686695. Epub 2015/12/22. eng.

15. Burghardt AJ, Issever AS, Schwartz AV, Davis KA, Masharani U, Majumdar S, et al. High-resolution peripheral quantitative computed tomographic imaging of cortical and trabecular bone microarchitecture in patients with type 2 diabetes mellitus. *J Clin Endocrinol Metab.* 2010 Nov;95(11):5045-55. PubMed PMID: 20719835. PubMed Central PMCID: PMC2968722.

16. Patsch JM, Burghardt AJ, Yap SP, Baum T, Schwartz AV, Joseph GB, et al. Increased cortical porosity in type 2 diabetic postmenopausal women with fragility fractures. *J Bone Miner Res.* 2013 Feb;28(2):313-24. PubMed PMID: 22991256. PubMed Central PMCID: PMC3534818.

17. Berg KM, Kunins HV, Jackson JL, Nahvi S, Chaudhry A, Harris KA, Jr., et al. Association between alcohol consumption and both osteoporotic fracture and bone density. *Am J Med.* 2008 May;121(5):406-18. PubMed PMID: 18456037. PubMed Central PMCID: PMC2692368.

18. Jugdaohsingh R, O'Connell MA, Sripanyakorn S, Powell JJ. Moderate alcohol consumption and increased bone mineral density: Potential ethanol and non-ethanol mechanisms. *Proc Nutr Soc.* 2006 Aug;65(3):291-310. PubMed PMID: 16923313.

19. Sommer I, Erkkila AT, Jarvinen R, Mursu J, Sirola J, Jurvelin JS, et al. Alcohol consumption and bone mineral density in elderly women. *Public Health Nutr.* 2013 Apr;16(4):704-12. PubMed PMID: 22800300.

20. Paccou J, Edwards MH, Ward K, Jameson K, Moon R, Dennison E, et al. Relationships between bone geometry, volumetric bone mineral density and bone microarchitecture of the distal radius and tibia with alcohol consumption. *Bone.* 2015 Sep;78:122-9. PubMed PMID: 25959415. Epub 2015/05/12. eng.

21. Lorentzon M, Mellstrom D, Haug E, Ohlsson C. Smoking is associated with lower bone mineral density and reduced cortical thickness in young men. *J Clin Endocrinol Metab.* 2007 Feb;92(2):497-503. PubMed PMID: 17077132.

22. Rudang R, Darelid A, Nilsson M, Nilsson S, Mellstrom D, Ohlsson C, et al. Smoking is associated with impaired bone mass development in young adult men: A 5-year longitudinal study. *J Bone Miner Res.* 2012 Oct;27(10):2189-97. PubMed PMID: 22653676.

23. Paccou J, Edwards MH, Patsch JM, Jameson KA, Ward KA, Moss C, et al. Lower leg arterial calcification assessed by high-resolution peripheral quantitative computed tomography is associated with bone microstructure abnormalities in women. *Osteoporos Int.* 2016 Nov;27(11):3279-87. PubMed PMID: 27325126. Pubmed Central PMCID: PMC5040512. Epub 2016/06/22. eng.

24. Kanis JA. Diagnosis of osteoporosis and assessment of fracture risk. *Lancet.* 2002 Jun 1;359(9321):1929-36. PubMed PMID: 12057569.

25. Stone KL, Seeley DG, Lui LY, Cauley JA, Ensrud K, Browner WS, et al. BMD at multiple sites and risk of fracture of multiple types: Long-term results from the Study of Osteoporotic Fractures. *J Bone Miner Res.* 2003 Nov;18(11):1947-54. PubMed PMID: 14606506.

26. Schuit SC, van der Klift M, Weel AE, de Laet CE, Burger H, Seeman E, et al. Fracture incidence and association with bone mineral density in elderly men and women: The Rotterdam Study. *Bone.* 2004 Jan;34(1):195-202. PubMed PMID: 14751578.

27. Sornay-Rendu E, Boutroy S, Munoz F, Delmas PD. Alterations of cortical and trabecular architecture are associated with fractures in postmenopausal women, partially independent of decreased BMD measured by DXA: The OFELY study. *J Bone Miner Res.* 2007 Mar;22(3):425-33. PubMed PMID: 17181395.

28. Stein EM, Liu XS, Nickolas TL, Cohen A, Thomas V, McMahon DJ, et al. Abnormal microarchitecture and reduced stiffness at the radius and tibia in postmenopausal women with fractures. *J Bone Miner Res.* 2010 Dec;25(12):2572-81. PubMed PMID: 20564238. PubMed Central PMCID: PMC3149820.

29. Vilayphiou N, Boutroy S, Sornay-Rendu E, Van Rietbergen B, Munoz F, Delmas PD, et al. Finite element analysis performed on radius and tibia HR-pQCT images and fragility fractures at all sites in postmenopausal women. *Bone.* 2010 Apr;46(4):1030-7. PubMed PMID: 20044044.

12

Assessment of fracture risk

EUGENE V MCCLOSKEY, WILLIAM D LESLIE
AND JOHN A KANIS

INTRODUCTION

Osteoporosis is operationally defined on the basis of bone mineral density (BMD) assessment, with recent refinements of the description focusing on measurements at the femoral neck as a reference standard (1). The WHO-defined T-score of −2.5 SD or lower, originally designed as an epidemiological tool, has been widely adopted as both a diagnostic and intervention threshold. The principal difficulty for fracture risk assessment is that this threshold has high specificity but low sensitivity, so the majority of fragility fractures occur in individuals with BMD values above the osteoporosis threshold (2). Over the last two decades, many risk factors have been identified that contribute to fracture risk, at least partly if not wholly independent of BMD; these include age, sex, a prior fracture (3), a family history of fracture (4) and lifestyle risk factors such as physical inactivity (5) and smoking (6). These and other factors have been combined in analyses of individual cohort studies to develop algorithms and scores to characterise future risk in an individual. Early examples include models derived from single cohorts such as the Study of Osteoporotic Fractures (SOF) (7) and the Epidémiologie de l'osteoporose study (EPIDOS) (8). Such independent risk factors used with BMD can enhance fracture risk assessment; additionally, the incorporation of risk factors that correlate with BMD (e.g. age, fracture, BMI) can also enfranchise fracture risk assessment in the absence of access to BMD tests. These were the considerations underlying the development of the most widely validated and utilised fracture risk assessment tool, the FRAX® tool, developed by the former WHO Collaborating Centre at the University of Sheffield.

FRAX: FROM BMD TO ABSOLUTE RISK

Risk factors for osteoporotic fractures and for hip fracture were identified from several unique population-based cohorts in diverse geographic territories using the primary individual data (9). In brief, approximately 60,000 participants, the majority women, had a baseline assessment documenting clinical risk factors for fracture, with approximately 75% also having BMD measured at the femoral neck. During approximately 250,000 patient-years of follow-up, 5000 incident fractures were recorded and enabled the examination of several individual risk factors for fracture and their inter-relationships with other risk variables, notably age and BMD. In order to combine several risk factors into a clinically useful prediction tool, the manner in which each risk factor expresses risk was standardised by determining the population relative risk for each risk factor, calculated as the risk of an individual with that risk factor compared with the whole population of the same age and sex (9,10). This approach enabled the combination of risk factors, following adjustment to take account of the contribution of one to another.

Several easily captured clinical risk factors, identified in a series of meta-analyses, were ultimately incorporated into FRAX (11). In the final model, the risk of fracture is calculated in men or women from age, body mass index (BMI) computed from height and weight and dichotomised risk variables comprising a prior fragility fracture, parental history of hip fracture, current tobacco smoking, ever long-term use of oral glucocorticoids, rheumatoid arthritis, other causes of secondary osteoporosis and daily alcohol consumption of 3 or more units daily. Femoral neck BMD can additionally be entered, either as a T-score or as the absolute BMD value along with the make of the scanner used in BMD measurement. It is important to note that in both male and female patients, the T-score should be derived using the NHANES III database for female Caucasians aged 20 to 29 years (12). The FRAX output is a 10-year probability of major osteoporotic fracture (hip, clinical vertebral, proximal humerus and distal forearm) and hip fracture alone. The use of absolute risk has been widely adopted in other disease areas, most notably in the assessment of cardiovascular risk, where the simultaneous consideration of smoking, blood pressure, diabetes and serum cholesterol permits the identification of patients at high risk in the next 5 to 10 years (13,14).

The use of absolute fracture risk has the potential to be applicable to both sexes, all ages, all ethnicities and all countries even though the incidence of osteoporotic fractures varies widely by age, sex, ethnicity and geography (Figure 12.1). An important distinction between FRAX and other fracture risk assessment tools [e.g. Garvan (15) or QFracture (16)], is the handling of death during follow-up. In the latter tools, death is usually a censoring event rather than treated as a competing risk, thus neglecting the possibility of dying before fracture. Probability of fracture, as determined by FRAX, also depends upon the

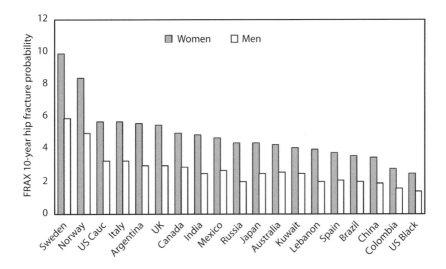

Figure 12.1 Demonstration of the wide variation in 10-year hip fracture probabilities in men and women in a sample of the country- and/or ethnicity-specific models available within FRAX. The example shown illustrates the probability in an individual at 70 years of age with a BMI of 24 kg/m² and a prior fracture.

risk of death, and when the risk of death is high the probability of fracture will decrease for the same fracture hazard.

In different regions of the world, the probabilities of fracture (17) and death vary markedly so that the FRAX models are calibrated to the known epidemiology of fracture and death. This assumes that the relative importance of the risk factors and their interactions are the same as in the original cohorts. At present, 63 country models are available, including 33 countries within Europe, and the tool currently provides coverage for over 80% of the global population (18). FRAX continues to expand, with country models being added or updated when adequate epidemiological data on fractures, particularly hip fractures, become available.

CAVEATS WITHIN THE CURRENT FRAX MODEL

Like all available clinical risk assessment tools, FRAX has several limitations that should be borne in mind when interpreting the results. These limitations have been addressed in detail elsewhere (19,20) and are only briefly summarised below.

Several of the clinical risk factors identified, for example alcohol consumption, glucocorticoid use and prior fractures, take no account of dose-response and provide instead a risk ratio for an average dose or exposure (21–23). In patients with a higher than average exposure, for example a daily dose of prednisolone of 10 to 15 mg, it should be recognised that the fracture probability is likely to be an underestimate; in the case of glucocorticoids, an estimate of this underestimation has been examined using data from the General Practice Research Database (GPRD) in the UK (24). At present the FRAX tool limits BMD inputs to that measured at the femoral neck, but other bone measurements can provide information on fracture risk; recent studies have examined the potential modification of the FRAX outputs by taking into account lumbar spine BMD or trabecular bone score, both of which contribute independently to fracture risk but appear to have limited overall impact on reclassifying individuals across assessment or intervention thresholds (25–28). Such approaches are probably best used in patients with fracture probabilities lying close to intervention thresholds.

Currently, a conservative assumption is made in the FRAX algorithm that the impact of causes of secondary osteoporosis on fracture risk is mediated fully by changes in BMD; thus when BMD is known, the secondary osteoporosis risk variable carries no additional weight in the calculation. A distinction is made between rheumatoid arthritis and other secondary causes, as there is good evidence that rheumatoid arthritis carries a fracture risk over and above that provided by BMD (29,30). Since the launch of FRAX, several other diseases have been identified as contributing to fracture risk independently of BMD, with probably the best example provided by type II diabetes mellitus. Several studies have shown that type II diabetes is associated with an increase in fracture risk (31,32) despite a higher mean BMD in such patients, in part reflecting the co-existing higher BMI. Nonetheless, the relationship with BMD and fracture risk is still maintained, i.e. patients with type II diabetes who fracture have a lower BMD than those with the disease who remain fracture free (32,33). In analyses from the Manitoba Cohort, FRAX calculated with BMD appears to underestimate fracture risk, confirming an independent contribution of diabetes to fracture risk (Figure 12.2) (34–36). It is likely that if similar evidence can be garnered from other populations and ethnicities, type II diabetes will become an independent input variable to future versions of FRAX. In the meantime, a number of potential interim solutions for use with the current FRAX algorithm have been proposed, including using the rheumatoid arthritis input to represent diabetes mellitus (37).

A frequently cited limitation of FRAX is the absence of a specific input for a history of falls or falling. This absence reflected a paucity of information on falls in the cohorts used to build FRAX as well as some uncertainty about the reversibility of risk attributable to falls by bone-targeted therapies (38,39). Since falls and fractures share many of the same risk factors, it would perhaps not be surprising to observe that baseline fracture probability, as calculated by FRAX, could also predict risk of future falls. This has recently been demonstrated in a prospective study of over 1800 elderly men in the MrOS Sweden cohort (40). In the proportion of the population with highest FRAX probabilities, set to equal the proportion with prior falls (16%), high compared with low baseline FRAX probability was strongly predictive of increased falls risk (HR, 1.64; 95%CI, 1.36 to 1.97) though somewhat weaker than the association between prior falls and future falls (HR, 2.75; 95%CI, 2.32 to 3.25). Importantly, the predictive ability of FRAX and prior falls were independent of each other, suggesting that even if a component of risk for future falls is captured by FRAX, this could be supplemented by specific information about prior falls. While further studies are

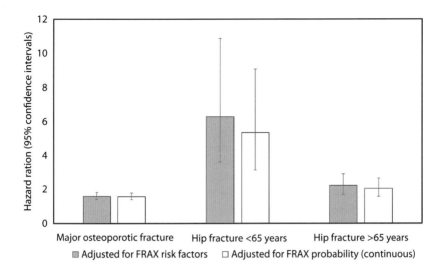

Figure 12.2 The association between diabetes and hip fracture risk and its independence from variables included in FRAX or FRAX probability itself. The increase in risk of major osteoporotic fracture is independent of age and sex, whereas the impact on hip fracture risk is greater at younger ages. (Derived from Gangregorio L et al. *J Bone Miner Res.* 2012 Feb;27(2):301-8.)

awaited, some guidance on the impact of the increased fracture risk associated with previous falls has been published (19,41), suggesting that FRAX probability of future fracture may be inflated by 30% (multiplied by 1.3) in a person with a history of falls.

INTERVENTION THRESHOLDS

The widespread uptake and availability of FRAX since its launch in 2008 has resulted in its inclusion in approximately 120 current guidelines across the world, 30 of which do not specify intervention thresholds (42). The incorporation of fracture risk assessment into clinical practice demands a consideration of the fracture probability at which to intervene, both for BMD testing (assessment thresholds) and treatment (an intervention threshold). Most current guidelines for osteoporosis recommend treatment for osteoporosis in individuals with prior fragility fractures, particularly in postmenopausal women; some guidelines restrict the prior fractures to those at the spine or hip (42). The recognition that treatment can be readily targeted to those with prior fracture (secondary prevention) underpins the approach to widen access to fracture liaison services (43–45). For those without prior fractures (primary prevention), or those without fractures of the spine or hip in particular guidelines, intervention thresholds based on absolute fracture risk have been derived using two broad approaches, namely the development of a *fixed threshold* probability that can be applied to men and women, irrespective of age, or the adoption of *age-dependent thresholds* where the fracture probability at which treatment is recommended is age-specific. Some guidelines have incorporated a hybrid of both fixed and age-dependent thresholds.

In a recent review, fixed probability thresholds in guidelines ranged from 4% to 20% for a major fracture and 1.3% to 5% for hip fracture (42). Importantly, over half of those espousing a fixed threshold utilized a threshold probability of 20% for a major osteoporotic fracture with most also proposing a hip fracture probability threshold of 3%; frequently the only rationale for such choices was that these were the thresholds adopted by the National Osteoporosis Foundation of the US (46). These thresholds were derived from a health economic assessment which was specific to the healthcare system, treatment costs and economy of the US at the time (47,48), so their adoption elsewhere needs to be treated with caution and ideally requires further justification. A health economic approach to defining fixed thresholds has also been undertaken in Switzerland; other approaches to defining fixed probability thresholds include the discrimination between fracture and non-fracture cases (Hong Kong), matching the prevalence of osteoporosis (China) and aligning with pre-existing guidelines or reimbursement criteria (Japan, Poland) (42). Some guidelines have chosen, perhaps somewhat inappropriately, to use a fixed threshold of fracture probability as a screening tool for bone density–defined osteoporosis (49,50); the sensitivity of this approach is less than other tools devised specifically for this purpose (51–53).

Intervention thresholds using age-specific fracture probabilities have been incorporated in a significant number of guidelines, including European guidance for postmenopausal osteoporosis and for glucocorticoid-induced osteoporosis. (54,55). The approach, first developed by the National Osteoporosis Guideline Group (NOGG) in the UK, is based on the rationale that if a postmenopausal woman with a prior fragility fracture is eligible for treatment, then at any given age, a man or woman with the same fracture probability but in the absence of a previous fracture (i.e. at the 'fracture threshold') should also be eligible (56,57). Given this premise, the fracture threshold automatically increases with age. In individuals in whom FRAX is calculated without BMD, subsequent reclassification rates by the inclusion of BMD are low and confined to individuals with values lying close to the intervention threshold (42,58,59). Thus NOGG additionally devised assessment thresholds around the intervention threshold to aid in the efficient use of bone densitometry, i.e. scans were targeted to those in whom there was a higher chance of moving across the intervention threshold in either direction, so that the scan was likely to influence treatment decisions (Figure 12.3).

Importantly, it has been shown that this approach, which was not based on cost-effectiveness was, however, cost-effective even when the analysis was conducted using a higher cost of oral alendronate than the current UK price (60). The NOGG approach has also been compared with previous guidance issued by the Royal College of Physicians, London (RCP) (61). Compared with the RCP strategy, NOGG identified slightly reduced numbers of women without prior fractures above the respective intervention thresholds, but these were at higher

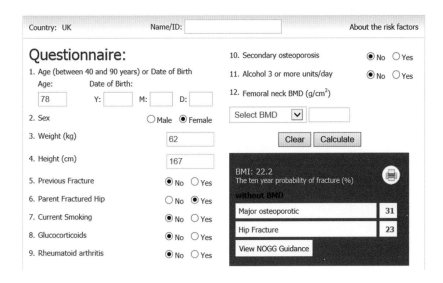

Figure 12.3 A screenshot of the UK calculator page on the FRAX website (www .shef.ac.uk/FRAX) showing the 10-year probabilities of major osteoporotic frac- ture and hip fracture in a woman aged 78 years, BMI 22.2 kg/m² and with a parental history of hip fracture. The NOGG button below the results connects the result, with guidance provided by the National Osteoporosis Guideline Group (www.shef.ac.uk/NOGG) (see Figure 12.4).

risk than those identified by the RCP strategy. A major benefit was a reduction in the number of BMD tests required using the NOGG guidance, resulting in significant economic dividends, with similar findings reported in studies from Belgium, Poland and the US showing that age-dependent thresholds were asso- ciated with greater dividends on budget impact (Belgium), cost/fracture identi- fied (UK) and improved sensitivity (US, Poland) than fixed thresholds (42). The recognition that women without prior fracture at older ages (>70 years) merited treatment at a higher threshold than women with prior fracture, resulting in inequalities in access to therapy, has recently led NOGG to adopt a hybrid model where the intervention and assessment thresholds are held constant from the age of 70 years upwards (Figure 12.4) (62).

This hybrid model reduces the disparity in fracture risk at older ages, increases treatment access and decreases still further the need for bone densitometry. The usage of the NOGG guideline is facilitated by a semi-automated linkage of the FRAX UK calculator web page to the NOGG web site to facilitate treatment deci- sions in the clinical setting (Figure 12.3) and this approach is widely used in the UK (63). Similar country-specific linkages are used in Finland, Lebanon and Romania.

10 -year probability of major osteoporotic fracture (%)

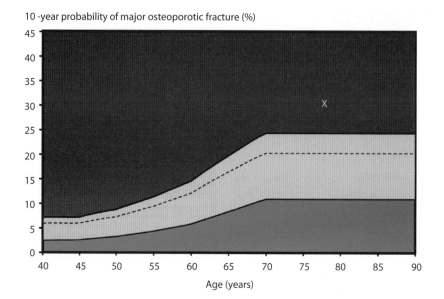

Age (years)

Figure 12.4 Example of the NOGG guidance output available within clinical practice. The major osteoporotic fracture probability is automatically placed on the 'traffic light' graph (shown as 'X' on the graph). Red indicates treatment, amber indicates consideration of a BMD measurement and green indicates lifestyle advice only and reassurance. If BMD is known, the graph consists only of red and green areas.

CONCLUSIONS

The use of tools that calculate absolute fracture risk is playing an increasingly important role in the clinical management of patients at risk of osteoporotic fracture. The FRAX tool should be considered as a platform technology on which to build as new validated risk indicators become available. Nevertheless, the present model provides an enhancement of patient assessment by the integration of clinical risk factors alone or in combination with BMD. Clinical utility requires the incorporation of such tools into clinical guidelines, and there is much evidence that this is being implemented; the setting of intervention and assessment thresholds within such guidance needs country-specific justification and support.

ACKNOWLEDGEMENTS

This chapter is substantially based, with permission, on McCloskey EV, Leslie WD, Harvey NC, Johansson and Kanis JA. Assessment of fracture risk with FRAX. *Endocrine Practice*. 2018.

REFERENCES

1. Kanis JA, McCloskey EV, Johansson H, Oden A, Melton LJ, 3rd, Khaltaev N. A reference standard for the description of osteoporosis. *Bone.* 2008 Mar;42(3):467-75. PubMed PMID: 18180210.

2. WHO. Assessment of fracture risk and its application to screening for postmenopausal osteoporosis. Geneva: World Health Organization; 1994.

3. Kanis JA, Johnell O, De Laet C, Johansson H, Oden A, Delmas P, et al. A meta-analysis of previous fracture and subsequent fracture risk. *Bone.* 2004 Aug;35(2):375-82. PubMed PMID: 15268886. Epub 2004/07/23. eng.

4. Kanis JA, Johansson H, Oden A, Johnell O, De Laet C, Eisman JA, et al. A family history of fracture and fracture risk: A meta-analysis. *Bone.* 2004 Nov;35(5):1029-37. PubMed PMID: 15542027.

5. Feskanich D, Willett W, Colditz G. Walking and leisure-time activity and risk of hip fracture in postmenopausal women. *JAMA.* 2002 Nov 13;288 (18):2300-6. PubMed PMID: 12425707.

6. Kanis JA, Johnell O, Oden A, Johansson H, De Laet C, Eisman JA, et al. Smoking and fracture risk: A meta-analysis. *Osteoporos Int.* 2005 Feb;16 (2):155-62. PubMed PMID: 15175845.

7. Black DM, Steinbuch M, Palermo L, Dargent-Molina P, Lindsay R, Hoseyni MS, et al. An assessment tool for predicting fracture risk in postmeno-pausal women. *Osteoporos Int.* 2001;12(7):519-28. PubMed PMID: 11527048.

8. Dargent-Molina P, Favier F, Grandjean H, Baudoin C, Schott AM, Hausherr E, et al. Fall-related factors and risk of hip fracture: The EPIDOS prospective study. *Lancet.* 1996 Jul 20;348(9021):145-9. PubMed PMID: 8684153.

9. Kanis J.A. on behalf of the WHO Scientific Group. Assessment of osteo-porosis at a primary health care level. Technical Report. WHO Collaborating Centre for Metabolic Bone Diseases. University of Sheffield, UK. 2007.

10. McCloskey EV, Johansson H, Oden A, Kanis JA. From relative risk to absolute fracture risk calculation: The FRAX algorithm. *Curr Osteoporos Rep.* 2009 Sep;7(3):77-83. PubMed PMID: 19723465.

11. Kanis JA, Oden A, Johnell O, Johansson H, De Laet C, Brown J, et al. The use of clinical risk factors enhances the performance of BMD in the prediction of hip and osteoporotic fractures in men and women. *Osteoporos Int.* 2007 Aug;18(8):1033-46. PubMed PMID: 17323110. Epub 2007/02/27. eng.

12. Looker AC, Wahner HW, Dunn WL, Calvo MS, Harris TB, Heyse SP, et al. Updated data on proximal femur bone mineral levels of US adults. *Osteoporos Int.* 1998;8(5):468-89. PubMed PMID: 9850356.

13. Goff DC, Jr., Lloyd-Jones DM, Bennett G, Coady S, D'Agostino RB, Gibbons R, et al. 2013 ACC/AHA guideline on the assessment of cardio-vascular risk: A report of the American College of Cardiology/American Heart Association Task Force on Practice Guidelines. *Circulation.* 2014 Jun 24;129(25 Suppl 2):S49-73. PubMed PMID: 24222018.

14. Hippisley-Cox J, Coupland C, Robson J, Brindle P. Derivation, validation, and evaluation of a new QRISK model to estimate lifetime risk of cardiovascular disease: Cohort study using QResearch database. *BMJ.* 2010;341:c6624. PubMed PMID: 21148212. PubMed Central PMCID: PMC2999889.

15. Nguyen ND, Frost SA, Center JR, Eisman JA, Nguyen TV. Development of a nomogram for individualizing hip fracture risk in men and women. *Osteoporos Int.* 2007 Aug;18(8):1109-17. PubMed PMID: 17370100. Epub 2007/03/21. eng.

16. Hippisley-Cox J, Coupland C. Derivation and validation of updated QFracture algorithm to predict risk of osteoporotic fracture in primary care in the United Kingdom: Prospective open cohort study. *BMJ.* 2012;344:e3427. PubMed PMID: 22619194. Epub 2012/05/24. eng.

17. Kanis JA, Johnell O, De Laet C, Jonsson B, Oden A, Ogelsby AK. International variations in hip fracture probabilities: Implications for risk assessment. *J Bone Miner Res.* 2002 Jul;17(7):1237-44. PubMed PMID: 12096837.

18. Oden A, McCloskey EV, Kanis JA, Harvey NC, Johansson H. Burden of high fracture probability worldwide: Secular increases 2010-2040. *Osteoporos Int.* 2015 Sep;26(9):2243-8. PubMed PMID: 26018089. Epub 2015/05/29. eng.

19. Kanis JA, Hans D, Cooper C, Baim S, Bilezikian JP, Binkley N, et al. Interpretation and use of FRAX in clinical practice. *Osteoporos Int.* 2011 Sep;22(9):2395-411. PubMed PMID: 21779818. Epub 2011/07/23. eng.

20. McCloskey EV, Harvey NC, Johansson H, Kanis JA. FRAX updates 2016. *Curr Opin Rheumatol.* 2016 Jul;28(4):433-41. PubMed PMID: 27163858.

21. van Staa TP, Leufkens HG, Abenhaim L, Zhang B, Cooper C. Oral corti-costeroids and fracture risk: Relationship to daily and cumulative doses. *Rheumatology (Oxford).* 2000 Dec;39(12):1383-9. PubMed PMID: 11136882.

22. Kanis JA, Johansson H, Johnell O, Oden A, De Laet C, Eisman JA, et al. Alcohol intake as a risk factor for fracture. *Osteoporos Int.* 2004 Sep 29. PubMed PMID: 15455194.

23. Delmas PD, Genant HK, Crans GG, Stock JL, Wong M, Siris E, et al. Severity of prevalent vertebral fractures and the risk of subsequent verte-bral and nonvertebral fractures: Results from the MORE trial. *Bone.* 2003 Oct;33(4):522-32. PubMed PMID: 14555255.

24. Kanis JA, Johansson H, Oden A, McCloskey EV. Guidance for the adjust-ment of FRAX according to the dose of glucocorticoids. *Osteoporos Int.* 2011 Mar;22(3):809-16. PubMed PMID: 21229233.

25. Leslie WD, Lix LM, Johansson H, Oden A, McCloskey E, Kanis JA. Spine-hip discordance and fracture risk assessment: A physician-friendly FRAX enhancement. *Osteoporos Int*. 2011 Mar;22(3):839-47. PubMed PMID: 20959961. Epub 2010/10/21. eng.

26. Johansson H, Kanis JA, Oden A, Leslie WD, Fujiwara S, Gluer CC, et al. Impact of femoral neck and lumbar spine BMD discordances on FRAX probabilities in women: A meta-analysis of international cohorts. *Calcif Tissue Int*. 2014 Nov;95(5):428-35. PubMed PMID: 25187239. PubMed Central PMCID: PMC4361897.

27. McCloskey EV, Oden A, Harvey NC, Leslie WD, Hans D, Johansson H, et al. Adjusting fracture probability by trabecular bone score. *Calcif Tissue Int*. 2015 Jun;96(6):500-9. PubMed PMID: 25796374. Epub 2015/03/23. eng.

28. McCloskey EV, Oden A, Harvey NC, Leslie WD, Hans D, Johansson H, et al. A meta-analysis of trabecular bone score in fracture risk prediction and its relationship to FRAX. *J Bone Miner Res*. 2016 May;31(5):940-8. PubMed PMID: 26498132.

29. Kanis JA, Johansson H, Oden A, Johnell O, de Laet C, Melton IL, et al. A meta-analysis of prior corticosteroid use and fracture risk. *J Bone Miner Res*. 2004 Jun;19(6):893-9. PubMed PMID: 15125788.

30. Orstavik RE, Haugeberg G, Mowinckel P, Hoiseth A, Uhlig T, Falch JA, et al. Vertebral deformities in rheumatoid arthritis: A comparison with population-based controls. *Arch Intern Med*. 2004 Feb 23;164(4):420-5. PubMed PMID: 14980993.

31. Schwartz AV, Sellmeyer DE, Ensrud KE, Cauley JA, Tabor HK, Schreiner PJ, et al. Older women with diabetes have an increased risk of fracture: A prospective study. *J Clin Endocrinol Metab*. 2001 Jan;86(1):32-8. PubMed PMID: 11231974.

32. de Liefde, II, van der Klift M, de Laet CE, van Daele PL, Hofman A, Pols HA. Bone mineral density and fracture risk in type-2 diabetes mellitus: The Rotterdam Study. *Osteoporos Int*. 2005 Dec;16(12):1713-20. PubMed PMID: 15940395.

33. Schwartz AV, Vittinghoff E, Bauer DC, Hillier TA, Strotmeyer ES, Ensrud KE, et al. Association of BMD and FRAX score with risk of fracture in older adults with type 2 diabetes. *JAMA*. 2011 Jun 1;305(21):2184-92. PubMed PMID: 21632482. Epub 2011/06/03. eng.

34. Giangregorio LM, Leslie WD, Lix LM, Johansson H, Oden A, McCloskey E, et al. FRAX underestimates fracture risk in patients with diabetes. *J Bone Miner Res*. 2012 Feb;27(2):301-8. PubMed PMID: 22052532. Epub 2011/11/05. eng.

35. Leslie WD, Morin SN, Lix LM, Majumdar SR. Does diabetes modify the effect of FRAX risk factors for predicting major osteoporotic and hip fracture? *Osteoporos Int*. 2014 Dec;25(12):2817-24. PubMed PMID: 25092059.

36. Majumdar SR, Leslie WD, Lix LM, Morin SN, Johansson H, Oden A, et al. Longer duration of diabetes strongly impacts fracture risk assessment: The Manitoba BMD Cohort. *J Clin Endocrinol Metab.* 2016 Sep 7:jc20162569. PubMed PMID: 27603908.

37. Leslie WD, Rubin MR, Schwartz AV, Kanis JA. Type 2 diabetes and bone. *J Bone Miner Res.* 2012 Nov;27(11):2231-7. PubMed PMID: 23023946. Epub 2012/10/02. eng.

38. McClung MR, Geusens P, Miller PD, Zippel H, Bensen WG, Roux C, et al. Effect of risedronate on the risk of hip fracture in elderly women. Hip Intervention Program Study Group. *N Engl J Med.* 2001 Feb 1;344 (5):333-40. PubMed PMID: 11172164. Epub 2001/02/15. eng.

39. Kayan K, Johansson H, Oden A, Vasireddy S, Pande K, Orgee J, et al. Can fall risk be incorporated into fracture risk assessment algorithms: A pilot study of responsiveness to clodronate. *Osteoporos Int.* 2009;20(12):2055-61.

40. Harvey NC, Johansson H, Oden A, Karlsson MK, Rosengren BE, Ljunggren O, et al. FRAX predicts incident falls in elderly men: Findings from MrOs Sweden. *Osteoporos Int.* 2016 Jan;27(1):267-74. PubMed PMID: 26391036. Epub 2015/09/24. eng.

41. Masud T, Binkley N, Boonen S, Hannan MT. Official Positions for FRAX(R) clinical regarding falls and frailty: Can falls and frailty be used in FRAX(R)? From Joint Official Positions Development Conference of the International Society for Clinical Densitometry and International Osteoporosis Foundation on FRAX(R). *J Clin Densitom.* 2011 Jul-Sep;14(3):194-204. PubMed PMID: 21810525. Epub 2011/08/04. eng.

42. Kanis JA, Harvey NC, Cooper C, Johansson H, Oden A, McCloskey EV, et al. A systematic review of intervention thresholds based on FRAX: A report prepared for the National Osteoporosis Guideline Group and the International Osteoporosis Foundation. *Arch Osteoporos.* 2016 Dec;11(1):25. PubMed PMID: 27465509. PubMed Central PMCID: PMC4978487.

43. Akesson K, Marsh D, Mitchell PJ, McLellan AR, Stenmark J, Pierroz DD, et al. Capture the Fracture: A Best Practice Framework and global campaign to break the fragility fracture cycle. *Osteoporos Int.* 2013 Aug;24(8):2135-52. PubMed PMID: 23589162. PubMed Central PMCID: PMC3706734.

44. Marsh D, Akesson K, Beaton DE, Bogoch ER, Boonen S, Brandi ML, et al. Coordinator-based systems for secondary prevention in fragility fracture patients. *Osteoporos Int.* 2011 Jul;22(7):2051-65. PubMed PMID: 21607807.

45. Javaid MK, Kyer C, Mitchell PJ, Chana J, Moss C, Edwards MH, et al. Effective secondary fracture prevention: Implementation of a global benchmarking of clinical quality using the IOF Capture the Fracture(R) Best Practice Framework tool. *Osteoporos Int.* 2015 Nov;26(11):2573-8. PubMed PMID: 26070301.

46. National Osteoporosis Foundation. Clinician's guide to prevention and treatment of osteoporosis. http://nof.org/hcp/resources/913. Accessed 9 Feb 2015.

47. Dawson-Hughes B, Looker AC, Tosteson AN, Johansson H, Kanis JA, Melton LJ, 3rd. The potential impact of the National Osteoporosis Foundation guidance on treatment eligibility in the USA: An update in NHANES 2005-2008. *Osteoporos Int*. 2012 Mar;23(3):811-20. PubMed PMID: 21717247. Epub 2011/07/01. eng.

48. Tosteson AN, Melton LJ, 3rd, Dawson-Hughes B, Baim S, Favus MJ, Khosla S, et al. Cost-effective osteoporosis treatment thresholds: The United States perspective. *Osteoporos Int*. 2008 Apr;19(4):437-47. PubMed PMID: 18292976.

49. U.S. Preventive Services Task Force. Screening for osteoporosis: U.S. Preventive Services Task Force recommendation statement. *Ann Intern Med*. 2011;154:356-64.

50. Scottish Intercollegiate Guidelines Network (SIGN). Management of osteoporosis and the prevention of fragility fractures. Edinburgh: SIGN; 2015. SIGN publication no 142. http://wwwsignacuk. Acccessed March 2015.

51. Crandall CJ, Larson J, Gourlay ML, Donaldson MG, LaCroix A, Cauley JA, et al. Osteoporosis screening in postmenopausal women 50 to 64 years old: Comparison of US Preventive Services Task Force strategy and two traditional strategies in the Women's Health Initiative. *J Bone Miner Res*. 2014 Jul;29(7):1661-6. PubMed PMID: 24431262. PubMed Central PMCID: PMC4117254.

52. Bansal S, Pecina JL, Merry SP, Kennel KA, Maxson J, Quigg S, et al. US Preventative Services Task Force FRAX threshold has a low sensitivity to detect osteoporosis in women ages 50-64 years. *Osteoporos Int*. 2015 Apr;26(4):1429-33. PubMed PMID: 25614141.

53. Kanis JA, Compston J, Cooper C, Harvey NC, Johansson H, Oden A, et al. SIGN Guidelines for Scotland: BMD versus FRAX versus QFracture. *Calcif Tissue Int*. 2016 May;98(5):417-25. PubMed PMID: 26650822. Epub 2015/12/10. eng.

54. Kanis JA, McCloskey EV, Johansson H, Cooper C, Rizzoli R, Reginster JY. European guidance for the diagnosis and management of osteoporosis in postmenopausal women. *Osteoporos Int*. 2013 Jan;24(1):23-57. PubMed PMID: 23079689. PubMed Central PMCID: PMC3587294. Epub 2012/10/20. eng.

55. Lekamwasam S, Adachi JD, Agnusdei D, Bilezikian J, Boonen S, Borgstrom F, et al. A framework for the development of guidelines for the management of glucocorticoid-induced osteoporosis. *Osteoporos Int*. 2012 Sep;23(9):2257-76. PubMed PMID: 22434203. Epub 2012/03/22. eng.

56. Compston J, Bowring C, Cooper A, Cooper C, Davies C, Francis R, et al. Diagnosis and management of osteoporosis in postmenopausal women and older men in the UK: National Osteoporosis Guideline Group (NOGG) update 2013. *Maturitas*. 2013 Aug;75(4):392-6. PubMed PMID: 23810490. Epub 2013/07/03. eng.

57. Compston J, Cooper A, Cooper C, Francis R, Kanis JA, Marsh D, et al. Guidelines for the diagnosis and management of osteoporosis in postmenopausal women and men from the age of 50 years in the UK. *Maturitas*. 2009;62(2):105-8.

58. Johansson H, Oden A, Johnell O, Jonsson B, de Laet C, Oglesby A, et al. Optimization of BMD measurements to identify high risk groups for treatment – A test analysis. *J Bone Miner Res*. 2004 Jun;19(6):906-13. PubMed PMID: 15190881.

59. Leslie WD, Morin S, Lix LM, Johansson H, Oden A, McCloskey E, et al. Fracture risk assessment without bone density measurement in routine clinical practice. *Osteoporos Int*. 2012 Jan;23(1):75-85. PubMed PMID: 21850546.

60. Kanis JA, Adams J, Borgstrom F, Cooper C, Jonsson B, Preedy D, et al. The cost-effectiveness of alendronate in the management of osteoporosis. *Bone*. 2008;42(1):4-15.

61. Johansson H, Kanis JA, Oden A, Compston J, McCloskey E. A comparison of case-finding strategies in the UK for the management of hip fractures. *Osteoporos Int*. 2012 Mar;23(3):907-15. PubMed PMID: 22234810. Epub 2012/01/12. eng.

62. McCloskey E, Kanis JA, Johansson H, Harvey N, Oden A, Cooper A, et al. FRAX-based assessment and intervention thresholds – An exploration of thresholds in women aged 50 years and older in the UK. *Osteoporos Int*. 2015 Aug;26(8):2091-9. PubMed PMID: 26077380.

63. McCloskey EV, Johansson H, Harvey NC, Compston J, Kanis JA. Access to fracture risk assessment by FRAX and linked National Osteoporosis Guideline Group (NOGG) guidance in the UK-an analysis of anonymous website activity. *Osteoporos Int*. 2016 Jul 20. PubMed PMID: 27438128.

13

Therapeutic approaches to bone protection in adulthood

ELIZABETH M CURTIS, MICHAEL R MCCLUNG
AND JULIET E COMPSTON

INTRODUCTION

Over recent decades, many effective treatments have been developed for osteoporosis. In this chapter, we review the existing pharmacological options to reduce fracture risk, document some of the emerging considerations regarding their use and describe novel therapies in development, which will further add to a comprehensive treatment armamentarium.

EXISTING PHARMACOLOGICAL TREATMENTS FOR OSTEOPOROSIS

Vitamin D and calcium supplementation

The presence of calcium as a major constituent of bone [a hierarchical structure built upon type 1 collagen matrix strengthened by calcium hydroxyapatite crystals (1)] clearly suggests its importance for maintenance of skeletal health. In most individuals, dietary calcium intake and endogenous vitamin D status are sufficient. However, there is evidence that supplemental approaches, particularly in individuals with inadequate calcium and vitamin D status, may benefit bone mass and reduce fracture risk (2–4). Both calcium and vitamin D have important roles to play in skeletal muscle; interaction between the skeleton and its associated musculature has been well documented, both through direct mechanical, and more recently, potential hormonal mechanisms. In skeletal muscle, calcium is closely involved in both neuromuscular signalling and in the regulation of intracellular actin and myosin fibres for muscle contraction and relaxation. Calcium is also key to the activation of glycolytic metabolism and mitochondrial energy metabolism, and there is evidence that vitamin D contributes to calcium uptake and regulation in muscle cells (5–7).

The role of vitamin D and calcium supplementation has been much debated in recent years, with several randomised controlled trials of either calcium alone or calcium in combination with vitamin D for fracture reduction, and subsequent meta-analyses aiming to elucidate the overall effectiveness of these interventions (8–10).

A large UK randomised controlled trial demonstrated that supplementation with either calcium, vitamin D or both for secondary fracture prevention at the population level appeared ineffective (11), although supplementation in high risk settings where deficiencies are expected, for example in nursing homes, may be beneficial (12). A recent individual patient data meta-analysis demonstrated that overall, there appeared to be a modest benefit for combined vitamin D and calcium supplementation for hip fractures, total fractures and probably vertebral fractures, but that there was no benefit for vitamin D alone (13). Although there has been discussion from one research group that excess calcium intake may be associated with increased cardiovascular risk (14), this has not been substantiated across many other studies. Indeed, it is reassuring to note that a recent individual-patient-data meta-analysis of the antifracture studies suggests that calcium and vitamin D supplementation in combination is associated with a relative reduction in mortality, which is not observed with vitamin D supplementation alone (15). Almost all of the randomised control trial evidence for the efficacy of anti-osteoporosis drugs comes from patients who were prescribed concomitant calcium and vitamin D supplementation; both should therefore usually be prescribed adjunctively with treatment for osteoporosis.

A recently published report by the European Society for the Clinical and Economic Aspects of Osteoporosis, Osteoarthritis and Musculoskeletal Diseases (ESCEO) and the International Osteoporosis Foundation (IOF) provided five main conclusions:

1. Calcium and vitamin D supplementation leads to a modest reduction in fracture risk, though has not been shown to be an effective public health strategy at the population level.
2. Supplementation with calcium alone for fracture reduction is not supported by the literature.
3. Side effects of calcium include gastrointestinal symptoms and renal stones.

4. Vitamin D supplementation, rather than calcium supplementation, may reduce fall risk.
5. The assertions of increased cardiovascular risk as a consequence of calcium and vitamin D supplementation are not convincingly supported by current evidence.

The authors therefore recommend that calcium with concomitant vitamin D supplementation is supported for patients at high risk of calcium and vitamin D deficiency and for those receiving treatment for osteoporosis (16).

Bisphosphonates

Bisphosphonates are synthetic analogues of the naturally occurring compound pyrophosphate and bind strongly to hydroxyapatite, inhibiting bone resorption by inactivating osteoclasts. The most commonly prescribed oral bisphosphonate is alendronate. If taken properly (in the morning with a glass of water, 45 minutes before food, drink or other medications and remaining upright for about 30–60 minutes after the dose), upper GI side effects are uncommon. However, for those who are unable to tolerate oral bisphosphonates, or in whom they are contraindicated (for example malabsorption or dysphagia), then an intravenous bisphosphonate such as zoledronate (given yearly in a dose of 5mg by infusion over a minimum of 15 minutes) is an alternative. Table 13.1 summarises the licensed indications for the currently available anti-osteoporosis medications.

Denosumab

Denosumab, a fully human antibody to receptor activator of nuclear factor kappa B ligand (RANKL) is a newer antiresorptive agent. RANKL, secreted by osteoblasts, is a major activator of osteoclastic bone resorption. Denosumab mimics the action of osteoprotegerin (OPG), the natural inhibitor of RANKL. It is

Table 13.1 European guidelines on the spectrum of anti-fracture efficacy of pharmacological interventions for osteoporosis

Intervention	Vertebral	Non-vertebral	Hip
Alendronate	+	+	+
Risedronate	+	+	+
Zoledronic acid	+	+	+
Etidronate	+	−	−
Ibandronate	+	+*	−
Raloxifene	+	−	−
Strontium ranelate	+	+	+*
Teriparatide	+	+	−
Denosumab	+	+	+

*Posthoc analysis in a subset of patients.

administered as a subcutaneous injection once every 6 months and its efficacy has been demonstrated in patients with renal impairment, although due consideration should be given to the possibility of underlying renal bone disease in chronic kidney disease (CKD) 4–5. Three-year fracture data show a 68% reduction in vertebral fracture and 40% reduction in hip fracture (17). Side effects are uncommon, but may include skin rash and skin infections, predominantly cellulitis, not related to the time or site of injection. Hypocalcaemia can also be a risk, particularly if the patient is vitamin D deficient or has renal impairment.

Strontium ranelate

Strontium, an element directly below calcium in group 2 of the periodic table, is combined with ranelic acid as a carrier to form strontium ranelate. It is taken as a single daily oral dose. Its mechanism of action remains a subject of research, but there is evidence that it increases bone strength by altering bone material properties. Administration of strontium ranelate leads to a substantial increase in BMD at the spine and hip, though part of this increase is artifactual, due to incorporation of strontium (which has a greater atomic weight than calcium) into bone. Studies have shown a 36% relative risk reduction in hip fracture over 3 years in osteoporotic patients (18). In 2013 a Medicines and Healthcare Products Regulatory Agency (MHRA) warning on strontium ranelate was issued due to increased risk of cardiovascular disorders (relative risk for myocardial infarction 1.6), in addition to the previously known risk of venous thromboembolic disease. Therefore its use is has been restricted to treatment of severe osteoporosis in postmenopausal women with high risk of fracture and in men at increased risk of fracture but with no cardiovascular or cerebrovascular disease. However, within this selected group of patients, particularly now that many individuals have undergone long-term bisphosphonate treatment, if available, strontium ranelate does still offer a useful alternative (19). This agent is not approved in the United States, and in 2017 Servier ceased its production.

Selective oestrogen receptor modulators (SERMs)

RALOXIFENE

Raloxifene is a selective oestrogen receptor modulator that has antiresorptive oestrogenic effects on the skeleton without the unwanted risks of oestrogen in the breast. Its use is also associated with a significant decrease in the risk of breast cancer. It has been shown to be effective in preventing post-menopausal bone loss and in preventing vertebral fractures. However there is no evidence that raloxifene prevents hip or nonvertebral fractures (20). Adverse effects include leg oedema, cramps, hot flushes and a two- to threefold increase in the risk of venous thromboembolism.

TERIPARATIDE

Teriparatide (recombinant human 1-34 parathyroid-hormone peptide) is the only agent in current widespread use with truly anabolic effects on bone. It is administered by subcutaneous injection in daily doses of 20 μg. It increases bone formation and produces large increases in BMD, leading to approximately a 70% reduction in the incidence of new moderate or severe vertebral fractures over 18 months of treatment, together with reductions in nonvertebral fractures (21). Side effects are uncommon but may include nausea, headache and dizziness; in addition, transient hypercalcaemia and hypercalciuria may occur. The use of teriparatide in the UK is currently limited to those older patients at highest fracture risk and who may have failed other therapies. Following teriparatide with a bisphosphonate or denosumab results in progressive increases in BMD (22,23).

COMBINATION THERAPY

The availability of pharmacological interventions with differing mechanisms of action has stimulated interest in the use of combination therapy with the aim of improving outcomes associated with monotherapy. Data are currently limited to changes in BMD, and the effects on fracture outcomes are unknown.

Combined anabolic and anti-resorptive therapy

PARATHYROID HORMONE PEPTIDES AND BISPHOSPHONATES

Combination therapy with parathyroid hormone (PTH) peptides (either PTH[1–84], no longer available in the UK, or PTH [1–34]: teriparatide) and bisphosphonates has been investigated in several studies. In the Parathyroid Hormone and Alendronate [PATH] study, combined treatment with PTH [1–84] and alendronate in postmenopausal women with low BMD produced similar increases in areal spine BMD to those induced by PTH [1–84] monotherapy, although a significantly greater increase in spine volumetric BMD was seen in the PTH [1–84] monotherapy group (24). In the hip, BMD showed no significant change in the PTH [1–84] monotherapy group but increased significantly in the combination group. Similar results were reported in longer-term studies comparing combined teriparatide and alendronate therapy with teriparatide alone, both in men and postmenopausal women with osteoporosis, although by 2 years spine BMD was significantly greater with teriparatide monotherapy than with combination therapy (25,26). In a study comparing combined teriparatide and intravenous zoledronic acid therapy with teriparatide or zoledronic acid monotherapy in postmenopausal women with osteoporosis, a more rapid rate of increase in spine BMD was seen in women receiving combination therapy than either monotherapy, although values after 1 year of treatment were similar in the combination and teriparatide monotherapy groups. In the hip, combination therapy was superior to teriparatide monotherapy in increasing BMD at all time points, with similar hip BMD increases in the combination therapy and zoledronic acid monotherapy groups (27).

TERIPARATIDE AND DENOSUMAB

In contrast to the effects of combination therapy with PTH peptides and bisphosphonates, co-administration of denosumab and teriparatide in postmenopausal women with osteoporosis resulted in greater increases in spine BMD than use of either drug alone (28). During 2 years of treatment, spine BMD continued to increase and remained significantly higher than in the monotherapy group (29). A similar pattern was seen in the femoral neck and total hip.

Collectively, these results indicate that combined PTH peptide and bisphosphonate therapy produces increases in spine BMD that are similar or slightly superior to those observed with PTH alone. At the hip, however, combination therapy is superior to PTH monotherapy and in the early stages of treatment PTH therapy may be associated with a transient decrease in hip BMD, probably as a result of increased cortical porosity. Combination therapy with teriparatide and denosumab, however, results in BMD changes in the hip and spine that are superior to those observed with either agent alone. The implications of these findings for fracture risk reduction are unknown. It should also be noted that in the studies discussed above, the vast majority of individuals were treatment naïve prior to therapy, and the results may not be applicable to patients previously treated with anti-resorptive therapy.

RARE SIDE EFFECTS OF BISPHOSPHONATES AND DENOSUMAB

Osteonecrosis of the jaw

Osteonecrosis of the jaw (ONJ) is a very rare occurrence in patients treated for osteoporosis with bisphosphonates or denosumab, with an estimated incidence of 1–90/100,000 years of exposure in patients taking bisphosphonates. Risk factors for its development include poor oral hygiene, dental disease, dental interventions, cancer, chemotherapy and glucocorticoid therapy (30). Patients taking bisphosphonates or denosumab should be advised to avoid invasive dental procedures if possible; for those in whom these are necessary, there are no data to indicate whether discontinuation of treatment reduces the risk of ONJ. During treatment, all patients should be encouraged to maintain good oral hygiene, have routine dental checkups and report oral symptoms such as dental mobility, pain or swelling.

Atypical femoral fractures

Atypical femoral fractures (AFFs), mainly affecting the subtrochanteric and diaphyseal regions of the femoral shaft, have been reported rarely in patients taking bisphosphonates or denosumab for osteoporosis. The estimated relative risk of these fractures in patients taking bisphosphonates varies widely, between 2- and 128-fold; the absolute risk is low, ranging from 3.2 to 50 cases/100,000 patient years. There is some evidence that the risk increases with duration of bisphosphonate therapy, and declines after its discontinuation (31–33). Atypical fractures occur with minimal trauma, may be bilateral and often exhibit poor healing. Radiological features include their origination as a transverse fracture line in the lateral cortex, often with localized periosteal and/or endosteal thickening, progressing to a transverse or oblique complete fracture with little or no comminution and medial beaking. There may also be generalised thickening of the femoral cortices. During treatment with bisphosphonates or denosumab, patients should be advised to report any thigh, hip or groin pain. If present, imaging should be performed and if an atypical fracture is present, the contralateral femur should also be imaged. Discontinuation of bisphosphonate or denosumab therapy should be considered, with switching to an alternative treatment if appropriate, and weight bearing should be restricted. Surgical intervention with intramedullary nailing is often required. Whereas these atypical fractures are rare, fragility fractures are common, and in high-risk patients the risk/benefit balance of bone protective therapy is strongly positive. Thus in a recent study from Denmark, long-term use of alendronate was associated with a 30% lower risk of hip fracture and no increase in the risk of fractures of the subtrochanteric femur and femoral shaft (34).

DURATION OF THERAPY

Bisphosphonates are by far the most commonly used bone protective therapy, and the optimal duration of treatment is the topic of much debate. The unique pharmacokinetic properties of bisphosphonates mean that they are retained in bone for some time after treatment is withdrawn, possibly translating into maintained efficacy for up to several years after withdrawal. This, together with concerns about the rare but serious potential side effects, discussed above, that may be associated with long-term bisphosphonate therapy, have led to the concept of 'drug holidays', in which bisphosphonate therapy is interrupted by periods generally ranging between 1 and 3 years and fracture risk subsequently reassessed before making a decision about further treatment. The evidence base for recommendations for long-term use of bisphosphonate and for drug holidays is limited, and currently there is no evidence on which to guide treatment decisions after 10 years of therapy (35).

Pivotal clinical trials of bisphosphonates have mainly been limited to 3 years, although there is reasonably strong evidence from extension studies that anti-fracture efficacy is maintained for up to at least 5 years of treatment. Withdrawal of treatment results in BMD loss after 1 to 3 years, depending on the bisphosphonate used, and data from the Fracture Intervention Trial Long-term Extension (FLEX) and the Health Outcomes and Reduced Incidence with Zoledronic acid Once Yearly (HORIZON) studies indicate that continuation of alendronate or zoledronic acid therapy beyond 5 and 3 years, respectively, is associated with reduced risk of vertebral fracture (36,37). Post hoc analyses from these studies suggest that women with low hip BMD (T-score $\leq$–2 to $\leq$–2.5), prevalent vertebral fracture or incident fracture during therapy are most likely to benefit from continued treatment (38,39). Based on these data, it is recommended that treatment review in people taking bisphosphonates should be performed after 3 to 5 years of therapy. In people aged $\geq$75 years with previous hip or vertebral fracture, incident fracture during treatment or treated with long-term oral glucocorticoids, continuation of treatment should be considered. In others, fracture risk reassessment using FRAX and BMD may be used to guide decisions about whether treatment can be stopped for a period of time (35,40). Importantly, discontinuation of therapy or drug holidays are not appropriate for non-bisphosphonate osteoporosis drugs (41).

NEW THERAPIES

Although several currently available drugs substantially reduce the incidence of vertebral and hip fracture, there is a need for therapies that are safer and more effective in reducing other fragility fractures. Three agents with novel mechanisms of action have recently completed Phase 3 fracture endpoint studies.

Abaloparatide

Abaloparatide is a synthetic 34 amino acid peptide that shares structural homology with parathyroid hormone–related peptide (42). It activates the same PTH-1 receptor as does teriparatide, but has a greater affinity for a particular G protein–dependent (GTPγS-sensitive) receptor conformation, called RG. In osteopenic rats, abaloparatide increased bone mass and strength while maintaining the normal mass:strength relationship (43–45). Increased risk of osteosarcoma was demonstrated in Fischer (F344) rats with near-lifelong treatment with abaloparatide similar to that observed with teriparatide (46).

In the Abaloparatide Comparator Trial In Vertebral Endpoints (ACTIVE) trial of 2463 postmenopausal women with osteoporosis, abaloparatide 80 μg/day subcutaneously induced smaller increases in markers of bone turnover than did open-label teriparatide 20 μg/day (47). However, after 18 months of therapy, the BMD increases in the lumbar spine were similar with abaloparatide and teriparatide, whereas the increase with abaloparatide in total hip BMD was larger. Abaloparatide significantly reduced the risk of vertebral fractures by 86% and of nonvertebral fractures by 43% after 18 months, effects that were not significantly different from teriparatide. However, the reduction in the risk of major osteoporotic fracture (70%) with abaloparatide was significantly greater than the statistically insignificant 33% reduction seen with teriparatide. Hypercalcemia occurred more commonly than placebo (0.4%) with both abaloparatide (3.4%) and teriparatide (6.4%). In a planned extension of the ACTIVE trial, fracture risk reduction observed with abaloparatide during the first 18 months of therapy were at least maintained when patients were switched to alendronate for an additional 6 months (48). Abaloparatide appears to be at least as effective as teriparatide and has a similar safety profile. The drug is now registered in the United States as a treatment for postmenopausal women at high risk of fracture. It will likely be used in the same patients for whom teriparatide is considered as appropriate therapy.

Odanacatib

Cathepsin K (CatK), a proteolytic enzyme secreted almost exclusively by osteoclasts, is the primary enzyme responsible for degradation of bone matrix collagen and other matrix-derived proteins and growth factors (49). Inhibition of CatK in rabbits and monkeys reduced bone resorption without reducing other functions of osteoclasts (50,51). As a result, bone formation was only transiently inhibited, in contrast to the marked and persistent decrease in bone formation with current anti-remodelling agents. This resulted in substantial increases bone mass, cortical thickness and bone strength. Several CatK inhibitors began clinical development. Because of off-target effects and other issues, only odanacatib, a highly specific inhibitor of CatK, entered into Phase 3 trials. Administered orally in a dose of 50 mg once weekly to postmenopausal women with low bone mass, odanacatib significantly increased BMD and reduced markers of bone resorption while bone formation markers returned to baseline values after about 2 years (52). The skeletal effects were quickly reversible upon stopping therapy. BMD in the lumbar spine and proximal femur increased progressively over 8 years, reaching average values of more than 12% and 9% from baseline, respectively (53). In patients who switched from bisphosphonates to odanacatib, BMD increased significantly (54). In the Phase 3 study in women with postmenopausal osteoporosis, odanacatib significantly reduced the risk of radiographic vertebral fractures by 54%, hip fracture by 47% and nonvertebral fracture by 23% (55). A significant relationship between nonvertebral fracture risk reduction and duration of therapy was observed; longer therapy resulted in greater risk reduction. Because of an unexpected increased risk of stroke in the treatment group compared to placebo, Merck chose to discontinue development of odanacatib (56). Thus our patients with osteoporosis will not have access to this very promising treatment that was conveniently administered, induced large and progressive increases in BMD and significant fracture risk reduction. It would have been an ideal agent to use in patients remaining at high fracture risk after 3 to 5 years of bisphosphonate therapy.

Antisclerostin therapy

Sclerostin, an osteocyte-derived glycoprotein that modulates bone formation by osteoblasts, is primarily regulated by mechanical loading; increased load reduces sclerostin secretion (57). By binding to LRP5/6, sclerostin inhibits the activation of the canonical Wnt signalling pathway, thus inhibiting bone formation. Patients with genetic deficiency of sclerostin exhibit increased bone formation resulting in high bone mass of normal quality (58). Sclerostin inhibition stimulates activity of osteoblasts and transforms bone lining cells into active osteoblasts (59). New bone is laid down on previously quiescent surfaces, a process called modelling-based formation, in contrast to the remodelling-based formation observed with parathyroid hormone analogues that require bone resorption prior to increasing bone formation. Antisclerostin antibody therapy in oestrogen-deficient rats and monkeys restored bone mass and strength (60).

Blosozumab and romosozumab are humanized antibodies that bind sclerostin with high affinity. Despite robust Phase 2 study results, the clinical development of blosozumab was halted. When administered subcutaneously, romosozumab induced prompt and substantial but transient increases in biochemical markers of bone formation, accompanied by a decrease in indices of resorption (61). BMD increased quickly, with changes from baseline reaching 11.6% in the lumbar spine and 4.1% at the total hip after 12 months of therapy. Continuing therapy for a second year increased BMD, although the increase during the second year was much smaller than had been observed during the first year, consistent with the effects of long-term therapy on bone remodelling (62). Upon discontinuing therapy, remodelling rates return to baseline, and the large increases in BMD fall to or toward pretreatment values.

In a Phase 3 fracture endpoint trial that enrolled 7180 women with postmenopausal osteoporosis, romosozumab 210 mg monthly for 12 months reduced the incidence of vertebral fracture by 73% (63). This effect was particularly evident during months 7 through 12 of therapy. During the second year of the study, all patients received open-label denosumab therapy. At the end of that year, vertebral fracture risk was reduced by 75% in patients who had received romosozumab during year one compared to the group that received placebo followed by denosumab. Clinical fracture risk was reduced by 36% compared to placebo after 12 months. The incidence of nonvertebral fracture was reduced by 25%, but this decrease was not statistically significant. Differences in fracture risk and responses to therapy were observed among geographic regions, with lower fracture risk and less response to treatment noted among patients in Latin America. Excluding the Latin American cohort, nonvertebral fracture risk was significantly reduced by 42%. It must be remembered that no therapy has been shown to reduce nonvertebral fracture risk within the first 12 months of therapy. Injection site reactions, usually mild, occurred in 5.2% of patients who receive romosozumab and in 2.9% of the placebo group. All oral adverse events and fractures of the femur were adjudicated by committees of experts. Two cases in the romosozumab group met the criteria for ONJ. One patient who had a history of pain in her femur at study entry experienced an atypical fracture of the femur 3.5 months after beginning therapy. No differences in the risk of cardiovascular endpoints were noted between the treatment and placebo groups.

Summary

The approval of abaloparatide and the anticipated availability of romosozumab will add to the anabolic choices for treating patients with osteoporosis. The Phase 3 studies with these two drugs are the first to demonstrate that the sequence of an anabolic agent for 12 to 18 months followed by a potent anti-remodelling agent is more effective in decreasing fracture risk than is starting therapy with an anti-remodelling agent (7,22). These studies provide strong justification for using an anabolic agent as first-line therapy in patients at high or imminent risk of fracture.

CONCLUSIONS

It is clear that there has been a massive expansion in the treatment options for osteoporosis in recent decades. Physicians are fortunate to have a range of therapies from which to choose, with the prospect of two further additions in coming years. However it will be several years before the next osteoporosis drug becomes available, since there are no agents in late Phase 2 or Phase 3 clinical trials for osteoporosis. It is likely that new molecular pathways will be identified, providing novel targets to evaluate. It is hoped that the field will have identified appropriate surrogates for fracture risk reduction so that trials with new agents can be performed more efficiently and with less cost. In the meantime, the focus of research must shift to developing clinical strategies though which our current treatment choices can be used more appropriately and more effectively. In addition, methods and tools, including the provision of adequate calories and protein as well as muscle anabolic agents such as selective androgen receptor modulators, will be developed with the objective of decreasing fracture risk by maintaining muscle mass and strength and reducing the incidence of falls.

REFERENCES

1. Seeman E. Structural basis of growth-related gain and age-related loss of bone strength. *Rheumatology (Oxford)*. 2008;47 Suppl 4:iv2-8.
2. Rozenberg S, Body JJ, Bruyere O, Bergmann P, Brandi ML, Cooper C, et al. Effects of dairy products consumption on health: Benefits and beliefs – A commentary from the Belgian Bone Club and the European Society for Clinical and Economic Aspects of Osteoporosis, Osteoarthritis and Musculoskeletal Diseases. *Calcif Tissue Int*. 2016;98(1):1-17.
3. Rizzoli R, Boonen S, Brandi ML, Bruyere O, Cooper C, Kanis JA, et al. Vitamin D supplementation in elderly or postmenopausal women: A 2013 update of the 2008 recommendations from the European Society for Clinical and Economic Aspects of Osteoporosis and Osteoarthritis (ESCEO). *Curr Med Res Opin*. 2013;29(4):305-13.
4. Ethgen O, Hiligsmann M, Burlet N, Reginster JY. Cost-effectiveness of personalized supplementation with vitamin D-rich dairy products in the prevention of osteoporotic fractures. *Osteoporos Int*. 2016;27(1):301-8.
5. Kuo IY, Ehrlich BE. Signaling in muscle contraction. *Cold Spring Harb Perspect Biol*. 2015;7(2):a006023.
6. Gehlert S, Bloch W, Suhr F. Ca2+-dependent regulations and signaling in skeletal muscle: From electro-mechanical coupling to adaptation. *Int J Mol Sci*. 2015;16(1):1066-95.
7. Rizzoli R, Stevenson JC, Bauer JM, van Loon LJ, Walrand S, Kanis JA, et al. The role of dietary protein and vitamin D in maintaining musculoskeletal health in postmenopausal women: A consensus statement from the European Society for Clinical and Economic Aspects of Osteoporosis and Osteoarthritis (ESCEO). *Maturitas*. 2014;79(1):122-32.
8. Tang BM, Eslick GD, Nowson C, Smith C, Bensoussan A. Use of calcium or calcium in combination with vitamin D supplementation to prevent fractures and bone loss in people aged 50 years and older: A meta-analysis. *Lancet*. 2007;370(9588):657-66.

9. Tai V, Leung W, Grey A, Reid IR, Bolland MJ. Calcium intake and bone mineral density: Systematic review and meta-analysis. *BMJ*. 2015;Sep 29;351:h4183. doi: 10.1136/bmj.h4183.

10. Bischoff-Ferrari HA, Dawson-Hughes B, Baron JA, Burckhardt P, Li R, Spiegelman D, et al. Calcium intake and hip fracture risk in men and women: A meta-analysis of prospective cohort studies and randomized controlled trials. *Am J Clin Nut*. 2007;86(6):1780-90.

11. Grant AM, Avenell A, Campbell MK, McDonald AM, MacLennan GS, McPherson GC, et al. Oral vitamin D3 and calcium for secondary prevention of low-trauma fractures in elderly people (Randomised Evaluation of Calcium OR vitamin D, RECORD): A randomised placebo-controlled trial. *Lancet*. 2005;365(9471):1621-8.

12. Chapuy MC, Pamphile R, Paris E, Kempf C, Schlichting M, Arnaud S, et al. Combined calcium and vitamin D3 supplementation in elderly women: Confirmation of reversal of secondary hyperparathyroidism and hip fracture risk: The Decalyos II study. *Osteoporos Int*. 2002;13(3):257-64.

13. Abrahamsen B, Avenell A, Anderson F, Meyer HE, Cooper C, Smith H, et al. Patient level pooled analysis of 68 500 patients from seven major vitamin D fracture trials in US and Europe 2010. *BMJ*. 2010 Jan 12;340: b5463. doi: 10.1136/bmj.b5463.

14. Bolland MJ, Avenell A, Baron JA, Grey A, MacLennan GS, Gamble GD, et al. Effect of calcium supplements on risk of myocardial infarction and cardiovascular events: Meta-analysis. *BMJ*. 2010; Jul 29;341:c3691. doi: 10.1136/bmj.c3691.

15. Rejnmark L, Avenell A, Masud T, Anderson F, Meyer HE, Sanders KM, et al. Vitamin D with calcium reduces mortality: Patient level pooled analysis of 70,528 patients from eight major vitamin D trials. *J Clin Endo Metab*. 2012;97(8):2670-81.

16. Harvey NC, Biver E, Kaufman JM, Bauer J, Branco J, Brandi ML, et al. The role of calcium supplementation in healthy musculoskeletal ageing: An expert consensus meeting of the European Society for Clinical and Economic Aspects of Osteoporosis, Osteoarthritis and Musculoskeletal Diseases (ESCEO) and the International Foundation for Osteoporosis (IOF). *Osteoporos Int*. 2017;28(2):447-62.

17. Cummings SR, Martin JS, McClung MR, Siris ES, Eastell R, Reid IR, et al. Denosumab for prevention of fractures in postmenopausal women with oteoporosis. *N Engl J Med*. 2009;361(8):756-65.

18. Reginster JY, Seeman E, Vernejoul MCD, Adami S, Compston J, Phenekos C, et al. Strontium ranelate reduces the risk of nonvertebral fractures in postmenopausal women with osteoporosis: Treatment of Peripheral Osteoporosis (TROPOS) Study. *J Clin Endo Metab*. 2005;90(5):2816-22.

19. Reginster JY, Brandi ML, Cannata-Andia J, Cooper C, Cortet B, Feron JM, et al. The position of strontium ranelate in today's management of osteoporosis. *Osteoporos Int*. 2015. 26(6):1667-71.

20. Ettinger B, Black DM, Mitlak BH, et al. Reduction of vertebral fracture risk in postmenopausal women with osteoporosis treated with raloxifene: Results from a 3-year randomized clinical trial. *JAMA*. 1999;282(7):637-45.

21. Neer RM, Arnaud CD, Zanchetta JR, Prince R, Gaich GA, Reginster JY, et al. Effect of parathyroid hormone (1-34) on fractures and bone mineral density in postmenopausal women with osteoporosis. *N Engl J Med*. 2001;344(19):1434-41.

22. Black DM, Bilezikian JP, Ensrud KE, Greenspan SL, Palermo L, Hue T, et al. One year of alendronate after one year of parathyroid hormone (1-84) for osteoporosis. *N Engl J Med*. 2005;353(6):555-65.

23. Leder BZ, Tsai JN, Uihlein AV, Wallace PM, Lee H, Neer RM, Burnett-Bowie SA. Denosumab and teriparatide transitions in postmenopausal osteoporosis (the DATA-Switch study): Extension of a randomised controlled trial. *Lancet*. 2015;386(9999):1147-55.

24. Black DM, Greenspan SL, Ensrud KE, Palermo L, McGowan JA, Lang TF, et al. The effects of parathyroid hormone and alendronate alone or in combination in postmenopausal osteoporosis. *N Engl J Med*. 2003;349(13):1207-15.

25. Finkelstein JS, Wyland JJ, Lee H, Neer RM. Effects of teriparatide, alendronate, or both in women with postmenopausal osteoporosis. *J Clin Endo Metab*. 2010;95(4):1838-45.

26. Finkelstein JS, Hayes A, Hunzelman JL, Wyland JJ, Lee H, Neer RM. The effects of parathyroid hormone, alendronate, or both in men with osteoporosis. *N Engl J Med*. 2003;349(13):1216-26.

27. Cosman F, Eriksen EF, Recknor C, Miller PD, Guanabens N, Kasperk C, et al. Effects of intravenous zoledronic acid plus subcutaneous teriparatide [rhPTH(1-34)] in postmenopausal osteoporosis. *J Bone Miner Res*. 2011;26(3):503-11.

28. Tsai JN, Uihlein AV, Lee H, Kumbhani R, Siwila-Sackman E, McKay EA, et al. Teriparatide and denosumab, alone or combined, in women with postmenopausal osteoporosis: The DATA study randomised trial. *Lancet*. 2013;382(9886):50-6.

29. Leder BZ, Tsai JN, Uihlein AV, Burnett-Bowie SA, Zhu Y, Foley K, et al. Two years of Denosumab and teriparatide administration in postmenopausal women with osteoporosis (The DATA Extension Study): A randomized controlled trial. *J Clin Endo Metab*. 2014;99(5):1694-700.

30. Khan AA, Morrison A, Hanley DA, Felsenberg D, McCauley LK, O'Ryan F, et al. Diagnosis and management of osteonecrosis of the jaw: A systematic review and international consensus. *J Bone Miner Res*. 2015;30(1):3-23.

31. Shane E, Burr D, Abrahamsen B, Adler RA, Brown TD, Cheung AM, et al. Atypical subtrochanteric and diaphyseal femoral fractures: Second report of a task force of the American Society for Bone and Mineral Research. *J Bone Miner Res*. 2014;29(1):1-23.

32. Gedmintas L, Solomon DH, Kim SC. Bisphosphonates and risk of subtrochanteric, femoral shaft, and atypical femur fracture: A systematic review and meta-analysis. *J Bone Miner Res.* 2013;28(8):1729-37.

33. Shane E, Burr D, Ebeling PR, Abrahamsen B, Adler RA, Brown TD, et al. Atypical subtrochanteric and diaphyseal femoral fractures: Report of a task force of the American Society for Bone and Mineral Research. *J Bone Miner Res.* 2010;25(11):2267-94.

34. Abrahamsen B, Eiken P, Prieto-Alhambra D, Eastell R. Risk of hip, subtrochanteric, and femoral shaft fractures among mid and long term users of alendronate: Nationwide cohort and nested case-control study. *BMJ.* 2016;353:i3365.

35. Adler RA, El-Hajj Fuleihan G, Bauer DC, Camacho PM, Clarke BL, Clines GA, et al. Managing osteoporosis in patients on long-term bisphosphonate treatment: Report of a task force of the American Society for Bone and Mineral Research. *J Bone Miner Res.* 2016;31(1):16-35.

36. Black DM, Schwartz AV, Ensrud KE, Cauley JA, Levis S, Quandt SA, et al. Effects of continuing or stopping alendronate after 5 years of treatment: The Fracture Intervention Trial Long-term Extension (FLEX): A randomized trial. *JAMA.* 2006;296(24):2927-38.

37. Black DM, Reid IR, Boonen S, Bucci-Rechtweg C, Cauley JA, Cosman F, et al. The effect of 3 versus 6 years of zoledronic acid treatment of osteoporosis: A randomized extension to the HORIZON-Pivotal Fracture Trial (PFT). *J Bone Miner Res.* 2012;27(2):243-54.

38. Black DM, Bauer DC, Schwartz AV, Cummings SR, Rosen CJ. Continuing bisphosphonate treatment for osteoporosis – For whom and for how long? *N Engl J Med.* 2012;366(22):2051-3.

39. Cosman F, Cauley JA, Eastell R, Boonen S, Palermo L, Reid IR, et al. Reassessment of fracture risk in women after 3 years of treatment with zoledronic acid: When is it reasonable to discontinue treatment? *J Clin Endo Metab.* 2014;99(12):4546-54.

40. Compston J, Cooper A, Cooper C, Gittoes N, Gregson C, Harvey N, Hope S, Kanis JA, McCloskey EV, Poole KES, Reid DM, Selby P, Thompson F, Thurston A, Vine N. National Osteoporosis Guideline Group (NOGG). UK clinical guideline for the prevention and treatment of osteoporosis. *Arch Osteoporos.* 2017 Dec;12(1):43.

41. McClung MR. Cancel the denosumab holiday. *Osteoporos Int.* 2016; 27(5):1677-82.

42. Hattersley G, Dean T, Corbin BA, Bahar H, Gardella TJ. Binding selectivity of abaloparatide for PTH-type-1-receptor conformations and effects on downstream signaling. *Endocrinology.* 2016;157(1):141-9.

43. Bahar H, Gallacher K, Downall J, Nelson CA, Shomali M, Hattersley G. Six weeks of daily abaloparatide treatment increased vertebral and femoral bone mineral density, microarchitecture and strength in ovariectomized osteopenic rats. *Calcif Tissue Int.* 2016;99(5):489-99.

44. Varela A, Chouinard L, Lesage E, Guldberg R, Smith SY, Kostenuik PJ, Hattersley G. One year of abaloparatide, a selective peptide activator of the PTH1 receptor, increased bone mass and strength in ovariectomized rats. *Bone.* 2017;95(Feb):143-50.

45. Varela A, Chouinard L, Lesage E, Smith SY, Hattersley G. One year of abaloparatide, a selective activator of the PTH1 receptor, increased bone formation and bone mass in osteopenic ovariectomized rats without increasing bone resorption. *J Bone Miner Res.* 2017;32(1):24-33.

46. Jolette J, Attalla B, Varela A, Long GG, Mellal N, Trimm S, et al. Comparing the incidence of bone tumors in rats chronically exposed to the selective PTH type 1 receptor agonist abaloparatide or PTH(1-34). *Regul Toxicol Pharmacol.* 2017;86(June):356-65.

47. Miller PD, Hattersley G, Riis BJ, Williams GC, Lau E, Russo LA, et al. ACTIVE Study Investigators. Effect of abaloparatide vs placebo on new vertebral fractures in postmenopausal women with osteoporosis: A randomized clinical trial. *JAMA.* 2016;316(7):722-33.

48. Cosman F, Miller PD, Williams GC, Hattersley G, Hu MY, Valter I, et al. Eighteen months of treatment with subcutaneous abaloparatide followed by 6 months of treatment with alendronate in postmenopausal women with osteoporosis: Results of the ACTIVExtend Trial. *Mayo Clin Proc.* 2017;92(2):200-10.

49. Duong LT, Leung AT, Langdahl B. Cathepsin K inhibition: A new mechanism for the treatment of osteoporosis. *Calcif Tissue Int.* 2016;98(4):381-97.

50. Duong LT, Crawford R, Scott K, Winkelmann CT, Wu G, Szczerba P, Gentile MA. Odanacatib, effects of 16-month treatment and discontinuation of therapy on bone mass, turnover and strength in the ovariectomized rabbit model of osteopenia. *Bone.* 2016;93(Sept):86-96.

51. Duong LT, Pickarski M, Cusick T, Chen CM, Zhuo Y, Scott K, et al. Effects of long term treatment with high doses of odanacatib on bone mass, bone strength, and remodeling/modeling in newly ovariectomized monkeys. *Bone.* 2016;88(Apr):113-24.

52. Eisman JA, Bone HG, Hosking DJ, McClung MR, Reid IR, Rizzoli R, et al. Odanacatib in the treatment of postmenopausal women with low bone mineral density: Three-year continued therapy and resolution of effect. *J Bone Miner Res.* 2011;26(2):242-51.

53. Rizzoli R, Benhamou CL, Halse J, Miller PD, Reid IR, Rodríguez Portales JA, et al. Continuous treatment with odanacatib for up to 8 years in postmenopausal women with low bone mineral density: A phase 2 study. *Osteoporos Int.* 2016;27(6):2099-107.

54. Bonnick S, De Villiers T, Odio A, Palacios S, Chapurlat R, DaSilva C, et al. Effects of odanacatib on BMD and safety in the treatment of osteoporosis in postmenopausal women previously treated with alendronate: A randomized placebo-controlled trial. *J Clin Endocrinol Metab.* 2013;98(12):4727-35.

55. McClung MR, Langdahl B, Papapoulos S, Saag KG, Bone H, Kiel DP et al. Odanacatib efficacy and safety in postmenopausal women with osteoporosis: 5-year data from the extension of the phase 3 long-term odanacatib fracture trial (LOFT). Annual meeting, American Society for Bone and Mineral Research, 2016, presentation number 1099.

56. Merck. Merck provides update on odanacatib development program. http://www.mercknewsroom.com/news-release/research-and-development-news/merck-provides-update-odanacatib-development-program. Accessed 28 June, 2017.

57. Li X, Zhang Y, Kang H, Liu W, Liu P, Zhang J, et al. Sclerostin binds to LRP5/6 and antagonizes canonical Wnt signaling. *J Biol Chem.* 2005;280(20):19883-7.

58. van Lierop AH, Appelman-Dijkstra NM, Papapoulos SE. Sclerostin deficiency in humans. *Bone.* 2017; 96: 51-62.

59. Kim SW, Lu Y, Williams EA, Lai F, Lee JY, Enishi T, et al. Sclerostin antibody administration converts bone lining cells into active osteoblasts. *J Bone Miner Res.* 2017;32:892-901.

60. Ominsky MS, Boyce RW, Li X, Ke HZ. Effects of sclerostin antibodies in animal models of osteoporosis. *Bone.* 2017;96(Mar):63-75.

61. McClung MR, Grauer A, Boonen S, Bolognese MA, Brown JP, Diez-Perez A, et al. Romosozumab in postmenopausal women with low bone mineral density. *N Engl J Med.* 2014;370(5):412-20.

62. McClung MR, Chines A Brown JP, Diez-Perez A, Resch H, Caminis J, et al. Effects of 2 years of treatment with romosozumab followed by 1 year of denosumab or placebo in postmenopausal women with low bone mineral density. ASBMR 2014 abstract 1152.

63. Cosman F, Crittenden DB, Adachi JD, Binkley N, Czerwinski E, Ferrari S, et al. Romosozumab treatment in postmenopausal women with osteoporosis. *N Engl J Med.* 2016;375(16):1532-43.

14

A lifecourse perspective on bone health and disease: Scientific and social implications

MARK HANSON, RUTH MULLER AND MICHI PENKLER

INTRODUCTION

Insights from research on the Developmental Origins of Health and Disease (DOHaD) point to the importance of the early life environment for bone development and later life risk of bone disease. The lifecourse concept further emphasises the role of different material exposures and social experiences across the lifecourse for continued bone formation and maintenance. From this point of view, bone health becomes a continuous process that involves multiple biological and social factors and which thus requires interdisciplinary investigation. In this chapter, we review the importance of DOHaD concepts for understanding bone health and introduce perspectives from the social sciences, such as 'embodiment', as important complementary tools for understanding bone health as a *biosocial* matter. We propose that such interdisciplinary approaches to bone formation and maintenance allow for a more holistic understanding of bone health and disease as well as for a more comprehensive perspective on the societal responsibility for bone health. We conclude that interdisciplinary collaboration is essential for adequately addressing the complexity of both the biological and the social processes involved in bone health and disease and for promoting more equitable translations of scientific insights into policy practices.

THE DEVELOPMENTAL ORIGINS OF HEALTH AND DISEASE AND THE LIFECOURSE CONCEPT

DOHaD was designated as a research field in 2003 when the International DOHaD Society was formed (https://dohadsoc.org). However, the concept dates from much earlier in the twentieth century when links between early development and risk of adult chronic, noncommunicable disease (NCD) were found. Kermack et al. (1) linked deprived living conditions characterised by infections and malnourishment in childhood with later premature mortality, and Forsdahl (2) made the link specifically with adult cardiovascular disease and found that this occurred even when the later adult environment was not deprived. Wadsworth et al. (3) subsequently reported an inverse association between birthweight, parental socio-economic status and systolic blood pressure in young men and women. The greatest contribution to the emerging DOHaD concept came from the series of epidemiological studies by Barker and colleagues from 1986 on (4–7), in which links were established between low birthweight, weight at 1 year of age and higher prevalence of hypertension, coronary heart disease, stroke and metabolic syndrome in adulthood.

Dörner and colleagues (see 8) extended the concept to developmental effects on later-life body weight, atherosclerosis and diabetes. His group were the first to use 'programming' (*Programmierung*) to describe such effects (9), a term adopted by Lucas (10), Barker (11) and many others. As the focus of the work became the link between low birthweight and later disease, the programming concept was taken to imply that the prenatal factors which led to low birthweight produced deterministically, albeit after a latency period of many years, the disease in an individual. This metaphor is more consonant with the genetic programme of development (12) than with the earlier observations which focused on early environment. Today, the effects of early environmental factors are thought more to induce different developmental trajectories which concern the magnitude and indeed sometimes the direction (13,14) of a response to a later challenge, such as living in an obesogenic environment. Moreover, the 'mismatch' concept (15) that risk of later disease would be greater if there were a disparity between the developmental and later adult environments – for example with socio-economic transition giving greater access to a calorie-dense and high-fat Western diet occurring between generations – was confirmed in both animal and human cohort studies (16).

Further refinements of the DOHaD concept stressed that it operates across the entire normal range of development, not just in association with extremes of development, and is therefore not a teratological process as Freinkel (17) and others had implied. This also brought DOHaD more into line with emerging ideas in developmental and evolutionary biology (see 18).

DOHaD AND PLASTICITY IN RELATION TO BONE

The role of developmental plasticity in mediating the effects of the early environment on later phenotype underlies contemporary thinking about DOHaD. In this respect, the skeleton provides a good example, as it begins to form early in gestation and provides a scaffold to which developing muscles are attached and grow. However, the skeleton remains one of the most plastic parts of the body, and the dynamic equilibrium between bone deposition and reabsorption continues throughout life, being affected by the loads placed upon it (19). The importance of vitamin D in these processes is discussed elsewhere in this volume. Lower levels of vitamin D are an issue during pregnancy (20,21), but also throughout life and especially in the elderly when hormonal changes reduce formation of new bone leading to osteomalacia, osteoporosis and increased fracture risk (see elsewhere in this volume). From this perspective, plasticity of the skeleton extends to a degree throughout life and does not conform to disposable soma or antagonistic pleiotropy theory (22,23). The concept of plasticity during ageing merits more attention (24).

The effects of poor nutrition, infection and environmental toxicants on skeletal growth of the fetus and child are well known, and reduced linear growth which leads to low stature, or 'stunting', remains a major concern in many low-middle income countries (25,26), being associated with a number of biological and social effects such reduced educational attainment, lifetime earning and longevity (27). Some of these effects point to social discrimination against stunted individuals in many societies (28). In addition, with the increasing adoption of Western diets and reduced levels of physical activity throughout the world, stunted children appear to be more likely to become overweight or obese as teenagers, especially young women (e.g. 29). While often considered a disease of the past, insufficient nutritional provision of vitamin D and low sunlight exposure are also associated with rickets in children, a condition seen in poor resource settings traditionally associated with poor nutrition but which is re-emerging in many parts of the world with urbanisation (30).

MATERNAL EFFECTS AND BONE DEVELOPMENT

The concept that aspects of the maternal phenotype, and her environmental exposures and experiences, can have important influences on the development of her offspring and may confer a Darwinian fitness advantage, is well established in evolutionary developmental biology (16,31). In humans, the effects of maternal diet during pregnancy, such as vitamin D levels, and other behaviours such as smoking, on the bone development of the fetus are well documented (see elsewhere in this volume). For human development, however, the concept of 'maternal constraint' of fetal growth – a process in which maternal factors limit the growth of the fetus during development (32,33) – has particular implications that are less widely known. Maternal constraint is greater in low-stature women, in first pregnancies and with a male fetus, which are risk factors for obstruction and complications such as obstetric fistula in low-resource settings (34). Greater constraint of fetal growth followed by more abundant nutrition in subsequent life might produce a greater degree of 'mismatch' between developmental experiences and the later life environment (15). This might increase the risk of noncommunicable disease in adults in these settings when economic development leads to adoption of Western diets and lifestyle.

There is also evidence for effects of maternal constraint in high-resource settings. In over 1 million births at 28 to 43 weeks' gestation from singleton pregnancies without congenital abnormalities in the period 2002 to 2008 in the Netherlands, the optimal size at birth for perinatal survival of the infant is substantially higher than the size at the 50th centile for the population (35), suggesting that even in such uncomplicated pregnancies maternal processes override to a degree those needed for survival of the offspring. The operation of maternal constraint of fetal growth in most pregnancies may partly explain the link between size and birth and later risk of NCDs across the entire birthweight spectrum.

A range of maternal behavioural factors also influence infant development of the fetal skeleton and can be interpreted in these terms. For example, in the Southampton Women's Study, a longitudinal prospective cohort, neonatal whole-body bone area and mineral content in both boys and girls was positively associated with maternal birthweight, and with the mother's current height and triceps skinfold thickness (36); as predicted, these neonatal characteristics were lower in first-born infants and in mothers who smoked. However, they were also negatively related to the mother's walking speed in late pregnancy, suggesting that such maternal exercise privileged her skeleton over that of her fetus.

UNDERSTANDING BONE HEALTH AS A BIOSOCIAL MATTER

The previous sections show that bones are an excellent example of an aspect of the body that remains plastic over the lifecourse and interacts with different factors in the environment. How we conceptualise these environmental factors is important on two levels. First, it influences our understanding of the aetiology of bone disease: for example, what do we identify as a cause of a certain bone health problem? Second, this in turn is important for the question of how to allocate responsibility for the bone health of individuals within a broader social context: who should act, and how, in order to improve the chances of good bone health for different members within society?

We propose that as lifecourse approaches become ever more important for understanding (bone) health, perspectives from the social sciences can contribute to conceptualizing environmental factors in the life sciences in ways that enhance both scientific accuracy and social impact. Such an interdisciplinary approach is well suited for exploring bones as a 'biosocial' matter: a physical substrate that is shaped by both basic biology and the social and material environments individuals experience across the lifecourse.

Within the social sciences, such an approach is referred to as the *embodiment* perspective. This perspective is interested in exploring how human bodies develop through actively engaging with their social and material surroundings (37,38) and change in response to the environments in which they live and the ways they live in them (39). From this perspective, our bodies tell the stories of our past experiences, some of which are visible to the naked eye while others can only be traced at the molecular level. Bone development and maintenance is, for example, influenced by eating habits, regular patterns of movement such as physical work and exercise (or the absence thereof) and exposure to sunlight. These are all activities with significant biological impact that are highly influenced by social, cultural and economic contexts (40–42). Paying close attention to these social and cultural factors shaping biological development can result in a more robust explanatory model of bone health and illness as well as more productive avenues for intervention.

Osteoporosis provides a good example of associated factors to which we might want to pay attention (see 41,42). Women are usually considered to have a much higher prevalence of osteoporosis than men. The condition is thus often framed as a 'women's disease' and explicitly and implicitly connected to biological sex difference and hormonal factors. While there appear to be sex differences in bone loss, the risk of osteoporotic fractures is more strongly associated with peak bone mass, which denotes that the highest level of bone strength humans usually reach is in their twenties to early thirties (41,43–45). Women tend to have, on average, a lower peak bone mass and hence less to lose before a critical low level is reached. While girls and boys have about the same bone mass until mid-puberty, subsequent bone development leads to an average greater bone mass in men (45).

The focus on the hormonal changes of menopause in the aetiology of osteoporosis has led research to largely focus on genetic and hormonal factors that may cause these gender differences in peak bone mass. However, there is evidence that physical exercise, nutrition and other lifestyle factors play an important role for bone formation too (41–43). It is thus probable that the different peak bone mass attained in young adult women and men is at least partly the result of different diets and exercise patterns between the sexes that are anchored in different societal gender roles for men and women (41). Diets and exercise patterns in return can also influence hormone levels and other molecular factors usually considered purely biological (41,46). This suggests that a disease that is usually conceptualised as the result of biological sex difference might be more complex and in part also the result of gendered social processes along the lifecourse. These social factors might present windows for possible intervention different from the paths currently pursued, for example enhancing gender equity with regard to nutrition and movement patterns in early to mid-life.

The example of a biosocial lifecourse approach to osteoporosis shows how an embodiment perspective can turn attention from explanatory models that locate the causes of health and disease exclusively within the interior of the body towards including the social environment as an important factor (39). Consequently, the social and the biological appear as inherently intertwined, and it becomes necessary to address them together.

Developing interdisciplinary collaboration that takes up this challenge is particularly important as lifecourse perspectives come to be extended beyond the life of the individual to include intergenerational effects. Increasingly, the prenatal period is considered of great important for later life health and disease (see Chapter 2 in this volume). For example, maternal vitamin D levels or maternal physical activity impact bone development during the fetal period and circumscribe chances for good later life bone health. As a consequence of this emerging knowledge, public health officials have been increasing their attention to maternal health during pregnancy and in the preconception period (47). This can be an empowering strategy that enables mothers to take their health and that of their offspring into their own hands. However, focusing public health interventions on mothers can also have unintended effects: it can heighten anxieties about responsible parenting among (already stressed) mothers and increase mother-blaming for all kinds of health outcomes in their children (48). Mother-blame can be particularly problematic if it is directed towards already socially disadvantaged women, such as low-income mothers or women of colour (49), who have often little access to the resources they need to live up to increasing standards of responsible motherhood.

Beyond mother-blame, the increasing focus on the prenatal period holds conceptual challenges that are of great societal significance. Expressions such as 'developmental programming' hold the danger of supporting determinist perspectives on biology that view individuals' lifecourses and health biographies as determined by early life experiences (50). The notion that some individuals might be programmed by adverse conditions in their early lives to express unhealthy phenotypes in later life and to develop disease might increase discrimination against such individuals. This is particularly problematic if such biological differences are framed as the shared characteristics of social groups defined by characteristics such as gender, ethnicity or social class. The proposition that the environment might be an intergenerational determinant of health, illness and ability of specific groups in society can come close to echoing eugenic positions of the past (50,51) that considered social position as both expressing and creating hierarchical biological difference. At the same time, it is important to point out that certain experiences and exposures that affect some groups in society more than others (the constraints of gender roles; racism; financial distress) can create and increase health inequalities. Here, the challenge for understanding bone health from a lifecourse perspective lies in developing biosocial accounts of bone growth that adequately capture the biosocial complexity of health inequality without succumbing to a determinist position (52).

CONCLUSIONS

A lifecourse perspective opens up a number of important avenues for understanding and addressing bone health in science and in society. Bone formation and maintenance can be understood as sensitive indicators of the wider social and material environment that an individual experiences across the lifecourse – from the womb to the tomb. These can reflect negative exposures and deprivation as well as positive stimulation and nourishment. The growth of the skeleton shapes adult stature, and stunted growth remains a major problem in low-middle income countries, as it is associated with a number of biological and social effects such as a greater risk of obesity and reduced lifetime earning. Beyond its dimensions, the structure of the skeleton is associated with risk of later osteoporosis and fracture. We used osteoporosis as an example to show how multiple influences across the lifecourse can influence disease risk. We pointed out how approaches from the social sciences that focus on social factors influencing risk (e.g. gender inequality in early to mid-life) can provide different avenues for disease prevention.

We have further outlined the potential scientific and social dangers that arise with a lifecourse perspective. Metaphors such as 'early life programming' can lead to determinist perspectives that view the chances of health in individuals, and possibly social groups, as predetermined by their early life experiences. Such a position not only fails to consider the ways in which bodies remain biologically plastic throughout life, but also bears the risk of increasing discrimination against already disadvantaged members of society. A responsibility falls on scientists and those who report on science to refrain from determinist language that suggests that health trajectories are predefined by intergenerational effects and early life experiences.

Bone health is an important issue for individuals as well as for society, and healthy bones constitute the basis for moving with ease and agility throughout life. However, health can also be a contentious issue that is in conflict with other important values in society. A lifecourse perspective emphasizes the importance of prenatal and early development, periods of life where individuals are highly dependent on resources and care provided by their parents. While this can lead to creating more support for parents facing difficult conditions, it can also lead to the policing of women's bodies during, and even before, pregnancy, and to a tendency to place blame on mothers. Here, health viewed as biosocial heritage that is passed from one generation to the next might clash with values such as gender equality and the freedom to make decisions about one's own body. Hence, addressing questions of bone health from a lifecourse perspective requires considering both its biological and social dimensions and consequences.

We thus argue for the importance of interdisciplinary collaboration between the life sciences and the social sciences for translating lifecourse perspectives on bone health into appropriate and equitable interventions in public health and other policy fields. Adopting a lifecourse approach reveals that some interventions to improve bone health more appropriately fall under the remit of social policy rather than health policy. Interdisciplinary collaboration can help to address this increasing complexity – both regarding how to understand the interaction of the social and the biological in this area of biomedical science adequately and how to translate this understanding into suggestions for responsible policy practices.

ACKNOWLEDGEMENTS

Mark Hanson is supported by the British Heart Foundation.

REFERENCES

1. Kermack WO, McKendrick AG, McKinlay PL. Death-rates in Great Britain and Sweden: Some general regularities and their significance. *Lancet.* 1934;223(5770):698-703.
2. Forsdahl A. Are poor living conditions in childhood and adolescence an important risk factor for arteriosclerotic heart disease? *Br J Prev Soc Med.* 1977;31(2):91-5. PubMed PMID: PMC479002.
3. Wadsworth ME, Cripps HA, Midwinter RE, Colley JR. Blood pressure in a national birth cohort at the age of 36 related to social and familial factors, smoking, and body mass. *BMJ.* 1985 Nov 30;291(6508):1534-8. PubMed PMID: 3933738. PubMed Central PMCID: 1418128.
4. Barker DJ, Osmond C. Infant mortality, childhood nutrition, and ischaemic heart disease in England and Wales. *Lancet.* 1986 May 10;1(8489):1077-81. PubMed PMID: 2871345.
5. Barker DJ, Osmond C, Golding J, Kuh D, Wadsworth ME. Growth in utero, blood pressure in childhood and adult life, and mortality from cardiovascular disease. *BMJ.* 1989 Mar 4;298(6673):564-7. PubMed PMID: 2495113. PubMed Central PMCID: 1835925.
6. Barker DJ, Winter PD, Osmond C, Margetts B, Simmonds SJ. Weight in infancy and death from ischaemic heart disease. *Lancet.* 1989 Sep 9;2(8663):577-80. PubMed PMID: 2570282. Epub 1989/09/09. eng.
7. Osmond C, Barker DJ, Winter PD, Fall CH, Simmonds SJ. Early growth and death from cardiovascular disease in women. *BMJ.* 1993 Dec 11;307(6918):1519-24. PubMed PMID: 8274920. PubMed Central PMCID: 1679586. Epub 1993/12/11. eng.
8. Dörner G, Rodekamp E, Plagemann A. Maternal deprivation and overnutrition in early postnatal life and their primary prevention: Historical reminiscence of an "ecologic experiment" in Germany. *human_ontogenetics.* 2008;2(2):51-9.
9. Koletzko B. Developmental origins of adult disease: Barker's or Dorner's hypothesis? *Am J Hum Biol.* 2005 May-Jun;17(3):381-2. PubMed PMID: 15849708.
10. Lucas A. Programming by early nutrition in man. *Ciba Found Symp.* 1991;156:38-50. PubMed PMID: 1855415.
11. Barker DJ. The fetal and infant origins of adult disease. *BMJ.* 1990 Nov 17;301(6761):1111. PubMed PMID: 2252919. PubMed Central PMCID: 1664286.
12. Jacob F, Monod J. Genetic regulatory mechanisms in the synthesis of proteins. *J Molec Biol.* 1961 1961/06/01;3(3):318-56.
13. Vickers MH, Breier BH, Cutfield WS, Hofman PL, Gluckman PD. Fetal origins of hyperphagia, obesity, and hypertension and postnatal amplification by hypercaloric nutrition. *Am J Physiol Endocrinol Metab.* 2000 Jul;279(1):E83-7. PubMed PMID: 10893326.

14. Gluckman PD, Lillycrop KA, Vickers MH, Pleasants AB, Phillips ES, Beedle AS, et al. Metabolic plasticity during mammalian development is directionally dependent on early nutritional status. *Proc Natl Acad Sci U S A*. 2007 Jul 31;104(31):12796-800. PubMed PMID: 17646663. PubMed Central PMCID: 1937546.

15. Gluckman PD, Hanson MA. *Mismatch: Why Our World No Longer Fits Our Bodies*. Oxford: Oxford University Press; 2006.

16. Hanson MA, Gluckman PD. Early developmental conditioning of later health and disease: Physiology or pathophysiology? *Physiol Rev*. 2014;94 (4):1027-76. PubMed PMID: PMC4187033.

17. Freinkel N. Banting Lecture 1980. Of pregnancy and progeny. *Diabetes*. 1980 Dec;29(12):1023-35. PubMed PMID: 7002669.

18. Gilbert SF, Epel D. *Ecological Developmental Biology: Integrating Epigenetics, Medicine, and Evolution*. Sunderland MA: Sinauer; 2009.

19. Ehrlich PJ, Lanyon LE. Mechanical strain and bone cell function: A review. *Osteoporos Int*. 2002 2002//;13(9):688-700.

20. Mahon P, Harvey N, Crozier S, Inskip H, Robinson S, Arden N, et al. Low maternal vitamin D status and fetal bone development: Cohort study. *J Bone Miner Res*. 2010;25(1):14-9.

21. Harvey N, Dennison E, Cooper C. Osteoporosis: A lifecourse approach. *J Bone Miner Res*. 2014 Sep;29(9):1917-25. PubMed PMID: 24861883. Epub 2014/05/28. eng.

22. Williams GC. Pleiotropy, natural selection, and the evolution of senescence. *Evolution*. 1957;11(4):398-411.

23. Kirkwood TBL, Rose MR. Evolution of senescence: Late survival sacrificed for reproduction. *Philos Trans Royal Soc London B: Biol Sci*. 1991;332(1262):15.

24. Hanson MA, Cooper C, Aihie Sayer A, Eendebak RJ, Clough GF, Beard JR. Developmental aspects of a life course approch to healthy ageing. *J Physiol*. 2016;594(8):2147-60.

25. Adair LS, Fall CHD, Osmond C, Stein AD, Martorell R, Ramirez-Zea M, et al. Associations of linear growth and relative weight gain during early life with adult health and human capital in countries of low and middle income: Findings from five birth cohort studies. *Lancet*. 2013;382(9891):525-34. PubMed PMID: PMC3744751.

26. de Onis M, Dewey KG, Borghi E, Onyango AW, Blössner M, Daelmans B, et al. The World Health Organization's global target for reducing childhood stunting by 2025: Rationale and proposed actions. *Matern Child Nutr*. 2013;9:6-26.

27. Hoddinott J, Alderman H, Behrman JR, Haddad L, Horton S. The economic rationale for investing in stunting reduction. *Matern Child Nutr*. 2013;9: 69-82.

28. Conrad P. *The Medicalization of Society. On the Transformation of Human Conditions into Treatable Disorders*. Baltimore MD: Johns Hopkins University Press; 2007. XIV, 204 S. p.

29. Kimani-Murage EW, Kahn K, Pettifor JM, Tollman SM, Dunger DB, Gómez-Olivé XF, et al. The prevalence of stunting, overweight and obesity, and metabolic disease risk in rural South African children. *BMC Public Health*. 2010 2010//;10(1):158.

30. Prentice A. Nutritional rickets around the world. *J Steroid Biochem Molec Biol*. 2013 7//;136:201-6.

31. Marshall D, Uller T. When is a maternal effect adaptive? *Oikos*. 2007;116(12): 1957-63.

32. Ounsted M, Scott A, Ounsted C. Transmission through the female line of a mechanism constraining human fetal growth. *Ann Hum Biol*. 1986 1986/01/01;13(2):143-51.

33. Gluckman PD, Hanson MA. Maternal constraint of fetal growth and its consequences. *Semin Fetal Neonat Med*. 2004;9(5):419-25.

34. Muleta M, Rasmussen S, Kiserud T. Obstetric fistula in 14,928 Ethiopian women. *Acta Obstet Gynecolog Scand*. 2010;89(7):945-51.

35. Vasak B, Koenen SV, Koster MPH, Hukkelhoven CWPM, Franx A, Hanson MA, et al. Human fetal growth is constrained below optimal for perinatal survival. *Ultrasound Obstet Gynecol*. 2015;45(2):162-7.

36. Harvey NC, Javaid MK, Arden NK, Poole JR, Crozier SR, Robinson SM, Inskip HM, Godfrey KM, Dennison EM, Cooper C; SWS Study Team. Maternal predictors of neonatal bone size and geometry: The Southampton Women's Survey. *J Dev Orig Health Dis*. 2010 Feb;1(1):35-41. doi: 10.1017 /S2040174409990055. PubMed PMID: 23750315; PubMed Central PMCID: PMC3672833.

37. Lock M, Farquhar J (eds). *Beyond the Body Proper: Reading the Anthropology of Material Life*. Durham NC: Duke University Press; 2007.

38. Ingold T, Gísli PI (eds). *Biosocial Becomings: Integrating Social and Biological Anthropology*. New York: Cambridge University Press; 2013.

39. Krieger N. Embodiment: A conceptual glossary for epidemiology. *J Epidemiol Commun Health*. 2005;59(5):350.

40. Agarwal SC. Bone morphologies and histories: Life course approaches in bioarchaeology. *Am J Phys Anthropol*. 2016;159:130-49.

41. Fausto-Sterling A. Bare bones of sex: Part I, sex & gender. *Signs*. 2005; 30(2):1491-528.

42. Fausto-Sterling A. The bare bones of race. *Soc Stud Sci*. 2008 2008/10/01;38(5):657-94.

43. Bonjour J-P, Chevalley T, Ferrari S, Rizzoli R. The importance and relevance of peak bone mass in the prevalence of osteoporosis. *Salud Pública México*. 2009;51:s5-s17.

44. Specker BL, Wey HE, Smith EP. Rates of bone loss in young adult males. *Intl J Clin Rheumatol*. 2010;5(2):215-28. PubMed PMID: PMC2897064.

45. Lang T. The bone-muscle relationship in men and women. *J Osteoporos*. 2011;2011:702-735.

46. Lock M, Kaufert P. Menopause, local biologies, and cultures of aging. *Am J Hum Biol*. 2001;13(4):494-504.

47. Waggoner MR. Cultivating the maternal future: Public health and the prepregnant self. *Signs*. 2015;40(4):939-62.
48. Richardson SS, Daniels CR, Gillman MW, Golden J, Kukla R, Kuzawa C, et al. Don't blame the mothers. *Nature*. 2014;512:131-2.
49. Mansfield B. Race and the new epigenetic biopolitics of environmental health. *BioSocieties*. 2012 2012//;7(4):352-72.
50. Kenney M, Müller R. Of rats and women: Narratives of motherhood in environmental epigenetics. *BioSocieties*. 2016 2016//(online first):1-24.
51. Hanson C. *Eugenics, Literature and Culture in Post-War Britain*. Abingdon: Routledge; 2012.
52. Hanson MA, Müller R. Epigenetic inheritance and the responsibility for health in society. *Lancet Diabetes Endocrinol*. 2017;5(1):11-2.

Epilogue

We hope that through the course of this book, the reader has become convinced of the value of a lifecourse approach to osteoporosis, and of the necessity to address both prevention at the public health level and the assessment and treatment of those individuals at highest risk.

Critically, the value of these approaches has been recognised and endorsed internationally, with the WHO and UN documenting the importance of the early environment for later chronic non-communicable disease, and novel approaches to risk assessment, such as the FRAX calculator, incorporated in a great many guidelines internationally.

So what does the future hold for this field? Again, one can consider this question at the level of the population and at that of individuals who are at high risk of fracture. Taking the latter scenario first, it is unfortunately very clear that despite huge efforts globally, there is still a substantial gap between the number of individuals who merit anti-osteoporosis therapy and the number who actually receive it. The need for improved coverage of individuals at high risk of fracture is the focus of an ongoing international task force, documented in detail in the 2016 International Osteoporosis Foundation World Osteoporosis Day report. We have the tools with which to assess fracture risk. We have mechanisms to identify individuals following an incident fragility fracture. We have effective medications to reduce the risk of future fracture. Indeed, we now have evidence that screening for fracture risk amongst older adults, using the FRAX calculator, leads to a reduction in hip fracture risk. The global imperative now is to implement the abilities that we have established to ensure that all those judged to be at high risk of osteoporotic fracture receive appropriate assessment and treatment.

There is an equally, if not more important (in that it affects a greater number of individuals) imperative to address bone health across the whole population from conception onwards, as supported by recent reports from the WHO and the UN. Although the majority of evidence in this area is observational, with novel randomised controlled trials such as MAVIDOS and SPRING, the evidence base to support early interventions to improve offspring health is being strengthened.

Further such intervention studies are required, ideally supported by mechanistic investigations, to definitively inform public health interventions aimed at improving bone health across the lifecourse. This work should be a global priority, and it is only with such investigations that we will be able to reduce the impact of this devastating disease in future generations.

Nicholas C Harvey
Cyrus Cooper

Index

Page numbers followed by f and t indicate figures and tables, respectively.